TEACH YOURSELF SEDUCTION

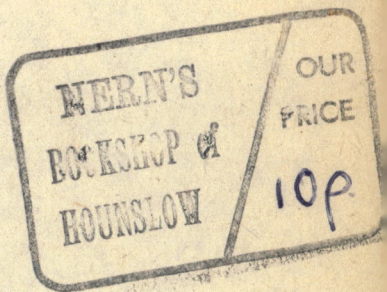

Teach Yourself
Seduction

Ruy Traube

NEW ENGLISH LIBRARY
TIMES MIRROR

First published in the United States of America by Belmont Productions Inc. in
December 1967
© 1967 by Script Associates

*

FIRST NEL PAPERBACK EDITION DECEMBER 1970

*

NEL Books are published by
New English Library Limited from Barnard's Inn, Holborn, London E.C.1.
Made and printed in Great Britain by Hunt Barnard Printing Ltd., Aylesbury, Bucks.

45000633 6

Contents

Seduction: The Spice of Life

A STEAK DINNER served by candlelight upon a fine table setting of linen, china and silver is far more appealing to the palate than a steak served at the end of a pointed stick. While it is true that both cuts of meat taste equally as delicious when one is hungry, nevertheless when one style of dining is served the same way night after night, the routine will soon jade the human appetite. Most people cannot for long tolerate monotony. It is human nature to crave variety in the mode of living. So it is with love and sex too. When love is "served" the same way every time, before long the appetite wanes, or at least becomes dulled. For this reason more than for any other perhaps, people seek other diversions in love. For most people, escape from humdrum love is impossible, yet they continually seek escape. Men and women develop roving eyes. They enter into fleeting affairs that eventually prove disappointing and sometimes lead to trouble. Few ever find utopian love, though they spend their lives looking for it. The reason they fail to find the "ideal" love is obvious. Love cannot be found—it must be created. It is an effort that must be worked at continually.

Like a garden that needs regular cultivation, love too is a garden that needs care and attention and occasional change of climate.

The wise husband and wife know only too well that romance and seduction are the spices of life and love. Nothing inspires renewed interest in love than the enthusiastic display of love itself. Whether this is demonstrated with a surprise gift or a novel way of lovemaking is of little consequence—the fact remains that the human psyche requires a change of pace if it is to remain vibrantly interested in life and love.

Too frequently, a man who is bogged down with work and the burdens of debt often neglects his wife and family. He soon loses his interest in lovemaking and eventually this leads to moodiness and apathy. Those around him live under a cloud of gloom. His entire outlook on life changes and he becomes embittered and disconsolate. The wife of such a man is wise if she continually strives to renew his interest in life—and love. She must be inventive at times, for when there is no money for other things, for the little luxuries of life such as the theater or dinner out, lovemaking is the only pleasure left that doesn't cost anything.

One happily married couple, though not well off financially, attribute the secret of their harmonious and contented life to what they call 'a game of seduction.' This couple, parents of three teenage children, make a game out of seducing each other. They never let a week pass without trying some new method of enticing each other sexually.

'It all started when I lost my job two years after we were married,' the husband stated. 'My wife saw that I was melancholy and had been losing interest in lovemaking. She tried to cheer me up when I left the house to look for a new job, but that didn't work. When I got home that evening—after a day of looking for employment, she greeted me at the door dressed in her apron, high heeled shoes, and nothing else. We laughed. She was particularly amused at the expression on my face. The kids were babies then, and one had not yet been born at the time, so we were more or less alone in the house. I made love to her in the kitchen.

'After that she tried to seduce me in a thousand different ways. I always found myself looking forward to coming home, not knowing what next to expect. She also doesn't know what to expect from me. I try—as I've always tried since that time too, to perk up her interest in me and keep it perked up. We've done some rather funny things and we've never regretted a single one. I might add that since we've always had so much fun together, the business of living and its trials and tribulations haven't mattered or come between us.'

This formula for happiness is a rather intimate and personal one, but it is successful because it works. If more people would adapt themselves to such a philosophy of living perhaps there would be less unhappiness and fewer divorces. The average human being resists change. He or she is apt to fall into a pattern of living that often becomes boring, dull, and mundane. But when a *habit* of having 'fun' in new and different novel ways is formed, life can be anything *but* dull and routine.

A poll of marriage counselors revealed that the details of seduction are often wanting for the simple reason that the sex lives of individuals are too private or intimate and few researchers are willing to take the time to ferret out the details of such practices. People are too reluctant to bare their souls, so to speak. But after many months of research, a number of interesting techniques of seduction have been collected. These are presented in the following text of this chapter. They are revealed in question and answer form, taken from the actual case histories and notes of practicing psychologists, psychiatrists, and marriage counselors.

How can I be 'sexy' toward my husband when I am not passionate by nature? I want to please him, but I can't seem to get with his sexy mood.

You are like millions of other women who are tired after a full day's work with your children and chores and or your careers; therefore you have convinced yourself you are *not* passionate by nature. No such thing exists. The truth is, you haven't really learned to 'turn yourself on'. You are weary at the end of the day, but not that physically exhausted that you cannot devote a few minutes to lovemaking. The trick is to 'think' seductively. Ask yourself how you can make yourself more attractive to your husband.

First, look at yourself in the mirror. Do you neglect your appearance? Do you happily greet your husband when he comes home from work? Do you look your best, with your face made up and your hair combed or brushed? Do you take the trouble to wear something feminine and alluring when you meet him at the door or do you wear an old pair of blue jeans or a frazzled housecoat that has seen its better days? The first step to take in becoming 'sexy' is to *look* sexy.

When he sees you through the eyes of a man who hungers for his wife, the 'sexiness' will naturally rub off. There is a certain magnetism which exists between a married couple, no matter how long they've been married. If the wife takes the time and the trouble to look seductive for her husband, she will succeed in keeping him interested—and, what's more, she too will become more passionate.

The fact that you want to please him is half the battle. Unfortunately there are those women who couldn't care less about seducing their husbands. They have lost interest in life and love and they seek escape by all means available to them. When this happens, when the children have grown and left the home, nothing personal or intimate is left. Such a couple left alone in their middle years often find themselves old before their time. They have acquired the habit of negligence. They have learned too late that they have taken each other for granted. When this happens they also find that they have taken for granted that they are 'too old' for youthful pursuits such as the practice of seduction 'fun and games.'

You ask how you can be 'sexy' toward your husband. This is not easy to answer because a lot of factors are involved. First, after you have learned to think 'sexy' and then after you have groomed and dressed yourself attractively and seductively, you must learn to lock your bedroom door when you and your husband are alone behind it—and *keep* it locked for as long as possible. You must learn to make your marriage bed a sanctuary, a refuge to which you and your husband may go in order to escape from the workaday world. You must learn to leave your troubles and cares locked *outside* that bedroom door while you and he are retiring inside. You must learn that time should stand still while you are together with your husband, and that your time together should not be hurried for any reason whatsoever.

Look around your bedroom and ask yourself if it is free of all the everyday things that make it less attractive and deter from its romantic appeal. Soft lights, ample pillows, the convenience of drinking glasses and perhaps some other effects which aid to your comfort and relaxation should be added to the room. The placement of mirrors in a provocative way can stimulate. A comfortable chair, and perhaps a soft rug will often work wonders when that door is closed behind you and your troubles are locked outside while you are alone with your husband.

Make it a practice never to mix pleasure with business. Taking your troubles to bed with you never solved them. Forget them and help your husband to forget them. Think sexy, be happy, and *think* happy —for then you will be truly happy. When you have done these things, and when it comes time to take him by the hand and lead him gently to the bedroom, your heart and his will sing with the joy of expectancy.

Many couples go through life without ever taking the time or the trouble to give themselves the time they

11

need to be alone—together. Many wives rarely—and sometimes never—take the initiative and show their husbands that they want *them* for a change. Frequently, many a marriage is saved when the counselor or psychiatrist suggests to a woman that *she* assume the initiative and ask the husband to make love to her. It has been found that most men feel they 'never get enough sex' because they always have to plead, argue beg and cajole their wives into surrendering. When a man must do this year after year, he naturally will begin to feel unwanted, rejected, and even unloved. Marriage and lovemaking is a two-way street. The wife *must* approach her husband sexually. She *must* take it upon herself to make herself 'sexy' by acting sexy. If she 'acts' that she is passionate, before long she will no longer have to 'act' that she is so, for she will develop a natural inclination to *be* passionate on her own initiative.

Remember, first look at yourself in the mirror. Where there is a will to improve your appearance, you will find the way to do so. Next, fix your bedroom up so it is more intimate. Make it look like a love nest instead of an everyday bedroom. Finally, take the initiative. Greet your husband with a hungry kiss, not a sisterly or motherly peck on the cheek. Show that you are anxious for him to make love to you, then lead him to your love nest and lock the door behind you. If you will do these things you will discover that you *can* be sexy toward your husband and that you *will* 'get with it' too.

My wife complains about sex all the time. She says I bother her too frequently and I ought to consider how tired she is after a hard day's work. She says that woman is the weaker sex, therefore they don't require sex relations as often as a man does. What can I do to make her understand that I don't get enough sex? I don't want to go to a prostitute or other women. I love her and I want her to satisfy me. She has never been very sexy.

From your question it is obvious that you have reached a point in life where you are contemplating extramarital affairs. Many men have reached such an impasse. Some eventually divorce their wives and marry other women. Some engage in relations outside marriage. And some sublimate their frustrated sex urges and bury themselves in work or other pursuits. But of these men, few take a positive attitude toward bettering their relations with their wives. Not only do they love the women to whom they are married, but they *want* to be loved in return. How then, can such women be reoriented in their attitudes and behavior toward their husbands?

First, there are many things to be considered. Some women have never been able to acclimate themselves to man's way of living. They believe that if they should show that they enjoy sex relations, their husbands would never let them alone. They believe that they would be in bed, morning, noon, and night, seven days a week. [Little do they know that such an idea is ridiculous, if not entirely impossible after a sustained length of time.] Moreover, there are some women who have been brought up to think that a display of sexual enjoyment is tawdry or unwholesome, if not indecent.

With the advent of so many hygienic devices, 'the pill,' and other contraceptive measures, there is no longer the fear of unwanted pregnancy to deter them; yet, women remain reluctant because it is sometimes inherent in their nature to be so. They have a way of separating 'love' from 'lust'. Some still believe that it is wrongful of man to 'lust.' There are even some who believe that intercourse should be indulged in *only* as a form of divine right or some other such hogwash. They are convinced of this and it takes years to make them

13

see how erroneous these views are.

When a man is confronted with the problem of making his wife understand that sex is nothing to complain about, he is bound to have a tough time convincing her otherwise with words. He must resort to ingenuity, if need be, to make her learn the truth. Sometimes a vacation away from home will give him the opportunity to seduce her and show her that sex can be fun. Sometimes, when nothing else is possible, a session of lovemaking at an odd hour of the day will suffice.

Then again, there are ruses and subtle strategems which may quickly change her way of thinking. For example, the wife who coldbloodedly turns her husband down time and again may be ripe for a rude awakening *if* her feeling of security and certainty is shaken. After all, the husband is usually the breadwinner. What will this woman think, and how will she react *if* she is given reason to suspect that her husband is attractive and desirable to other women?

At times, a smear of lipstick on a shirt collar, or even a phone call from a female 'wrong number caller' may do the trick. At other times, more drastic action must be resorted to—but with careful premeditation, for this sort of thing is dangerous. The ruse may backfire.

Another technique is to feign jealousy, to act as if you were suspicious of *her*. If she is characteristically defensive by nature her reaction may be such that she will do everything in her power to allay any fears or doubts about her fidelity. Of course, subtlety is the keynote again, and such accusations must not be made openly; instead they must be suggested.

When a woman has been found to be physically healthy and normal and there are no reasons why she should find sex relations unpleasant, the man whose wife complains about having sex relations must reflect carefully about his past relationship with his wife.

14

First, he must consider if he has ever given her any reason to mistrust him. Many women have grown up with the conviction that all men are cheats and cannot be true to one woman; therefore, they believe they should keep their husbands at bay in order to punish them for their imagined transgressions. Other women may feel that man must be continually kept sexually unsatisfied in order to keep them coming back for more —and to keep them at home.

And still other women have grown to dislike intercourse because their husbands have *not* been considerate enough of them. By considerate we of course mean in *all* ways. Do you help her with the little chores at home? Do you volunteer to take out the garbage or help her move the furniture, or do you curse and grumble and balk at every little thing she asks you to do? Little grains of sand make the mighty beach and erode the great rocks—so do the little unpleasantries one exhibits toward his loved ones. A little act of courtesy, like helping your wife out of the car will go a long way toward boosting her ego and elevating her esteem for you.

At parties and social gatherings do you show that you love her and are chivalrous toward her in front of others, or do you sometimes embarrass her or treat her without respect which in some way humiliates her before those she counts among her friends and acquaintances? The chances are you may have 'rubbed her the wrong way' more than once without knowing it. When you have done this unthinkingly, she will quite naturally rebel against you and in some way, attempt to pay you back. She will reject you in bed, she may reject you in other ways too.

It is not easy for anyone to change; but life and love are a matter of giving and giving and giving before one receives. If you are that frustrated sexually, and your wife continually harangues you about your constant need for sex relations, you *must*, we repeat *must*, go

15

about winning her over to your way of thinking and doing by a concerted, unrelenting campaign of chivalry.

Little things do mean a lot to women!

Think back to when you were courting her, to the days before you were married. Try to recapture your mental state then and revive that way of thinking and doing. Little acts of kindness, of chivalrous behavior go a long way. The woman whose husband literally jumps to see to her comfort is made to feel like a queen when she is alone – and when she is with her friends. This campaign, when sincerely undertaken, will achieve a small miracle in a relatively short period of time. It may take her time to come round to responding to your sexual advances, but when she does it will be well worth the effort. Then, when you feel you've made some progress, *continue* without letup your program of showering her with kindness and attention. Of course, don't overdo it. But be reasonable and patient and before long you will conquer her. This is the way to recapture the love of a woman who has begun to take you for granted and treat you like a mealticket instead of a lover and mate.

The use of gifts, no matter how trifling or inexpensive, are extremely helpful too. When one cannot afford a box of candy, a ten cent bar of her favourite sweet may do just as well – the point is, you *remembered* her. You were thoughtful, and you cared enough to show her that you think of her.

Greeting cards of all sorts are extremely valuable when wooing your wife. But be sure they are chosen in good taste and reflect what you mean. Tell her you love her in as many ways that you can – but tell her.

The woman who asks her husband if he loves her is asking because she inwardly feels insecure. Age is creeping up on her and she needs constant reassurance that she is as beautiful and lovable and desirable as ever. If your wife has ever asked you if you still loved

16

her, you may be sure that she has had her doubts. Think. If she *has* asked, then you must tell her how much you love her and appreciate her.

Nothing is more harmful to the relationship between a man and a woman than tactlessness. If you complain about the way she's set the table or if you make a face of displeasure when you taste her coffee, you are undermining her feelings toward you. More women than one can count have rejected their husband's sexual advances because the men were tactless enough to be uncomplimentary about something they have taken the trouble to do for them.

Woman is a paradox of behavior. She is more emotional and sensitive than man. The least little thing will unsettle a woman's attitude toward her husband; conversely, the smallest act done to assuage her ego will make her heart go out to her husband.

When tired, not completely and utterly exhausted, but normally tired, it takes a small amount of effort to relax her and help her unwind before she can be considered responsive to sexual advances. Perhaps a glass of milk or a cocktail may do more than words – especially when you bring it to her after she is in bed. The little touch of kindness, of attention, goes a long way toward rejuvenating her depleted energies. She has had a tough and trying day and she does not want to wrestle or argue with you. She wants to unwind and relax. She wants to be caressed and petted and she'll respond quickly enough when you show her you understand.

The woman who is tired will always show a lack of enthusiasm for the love act if her husband foolishly and uncouthly tells her he wants to have intercourse. But, the woman who is tired will always be stirred when her husband approaches her like a lover. The response will be mutual *provided* he works up to it, provided he awakens her interest in lovemaking by caressing her and kissing her, *not* by saying, 'Come on, let's do it.'

Those words, or others to that effect, have a dampening reaction on the feminine libido. When a woman hears them she unconsciously reacts by repulsing such an advance. She hears such sordid words and they *sound* sordid to her; she feels she is being *used*, not loved. She is willing, most of the time of course, to satisfy her husband; but she is *un*willing to respond to him because she has been made to feel that all he wants to do is satisfy his lust on her.

Of course woman is the weaker sex – but when it comes to the love act, she doesn't have to be as strong as the man in order to respond. When she lies back and lets him love her, and if he is considerate and understanding and patient enough, she will respond. She wants to feel that she is the most important person on earth to her husband, just as he wants to feel likewise with regard to his wife's feeling about him. When this is understood, and man overcomes his boyish frankness and resorts to the more manly subtleties of the lovemaking approach, he will find that his wife will respond – and eagerly – practically every time.

Heaven on earth can be discovered by two people when they are in each others' arms *when* each is certain that the other truly does care and wholeheartedly loves and needs them.

More marriages are broken up by third parties who do know the artful finesse of lovemaking than there are marriages which are saved by husbands and wives who fail to practice what they already know. Marriage, as with all things, is something which must be worked at constantly. Romance is necessary to lovemaking just as food is necessary to the sustaining of life. Without romance, there can be no lovemaking. Love then becomes a mechanical process. No married couple – in fact, no healthy man or woman anywhere can sustain their lovelife without romance and without the responsive embraces of their partners. True compatibility begins when each partner is able to mutually share the enjoyment of sexual fulfillment. Perversity exists when one continually takes advantage of the other partner. Instead of love, slavery exists then, for lovemaking requires that both man and woman give and take of and for themselves. The most profound feeling of all takes place when the human body is giving and receiving all at the same moment. The thrill of watching the reaction of an ecstatic moment being enjoyed on the face and in the body of a loved one is the greatest single thrill man can enjoy. Those who fail to develop their abilities to achieve this aim, also fail to live their lives to the fullest.

The woman who claims she has never been very 'sexy' more often than not has *not* been made to feel 'sexy' by her husband. When she complains that she is 'too tired' and 'I'm not sexy tonight' she is stating the truth: she is tired of the way her husband approaches her, and her libido hasn't been awakened enough to make her 'feel sexy'. It's as simple as that. It's therefore the man's job to overcome these feelings. He can revive her vitality by awakening her energy with proper seduction techniques. He can make her feel 'sexy' by making her desire him. When he uses commonsense and does the things which have just been outlined here to reply to the question asked several pages back, he will find that not only will his wife respond to his sexual advances, but that he will also find the love act to be more thrilling.

Too many men fail to realize that when they have set their caps for women outside of the boundary of marriage, they spend ninety-nine percent of their time courting and wooing their intentioned conquests and only one percent of the time in sexual intercourse. They fail to realize that they must spend weeks, and sometimes months, pursuing their game. They must shower them with gifts, lure them out on dates to expensive places and so forth before the opportunities arise when they can lure them into a bedroom. Is the chase worth the prize? Is the effort worth the end result? Surprisingly many men think so, because they continuously pursue women – with but one thought in mind – to get them in bed. Man is a charmer when he wants to be – he can conquer any female he sets his mind to conquer, provided he is subtle enough and relentless enough, and provided she is attracted to him. But after such men have wooed and won their fair damsels, how many of them continue the courting game after they have been married? Is it any wonder then, why so many desirable young women lose interest in matters of love and sex?

By today's standards of society, man is the hunter and woman the hunted. Why then should man cease his pursuit of woman as soon as he places a ring on her finger? Conversely, many women also cease their efforts to lure their husbands once they have been married. Does a marriage license mean to these people that a need no longer exists whereby they must be attractive to their mates? Does this mean also that they no longer have to go to such lengths to *seduce* their mates and keep them sexually interested?

Of course not.

As it has been stated previously, human beings are creatures of habit. They are prone to fall into patterned ruts of behaviour. They find it a lot easier to plod along in a routine way of living than to seek new and more interesting modes of living. When the novelty of marriage wears off, monotony sets in. Boredom follows monotony. Then greener pastures loom. The girl at the office suddenly looks alluring and enticing to the bored husband. The insurance man or the milkman or the boss [if she is a working wife] suddenly looks dashing and romantic and attractive to the bored wife. Opportunity arises and another marriage is on its way to the divorce courts.

Why do men and women cheat on each other when their marriages seemingly have so much to offer? It is needless to answer such a question except to say that it is usually the fault of either or both of the marriage partners.

There are of course extenuating circumstances which cause extramarital affairs; but these usually are fostered by basically insecure individuals who are so emotionally immature or disturbed that they are impelled to look for trouble elsewhere because their husbands or wives are 'on' to them. The emotionally immature husband who feels he must prove himself a lady killer is a man who usually cannot be true to one woman as long as he remains emotionally immature. The vain, emotionally distraught or immature young wife must also prove to herself and to the world that she is able to seduce the attractive men who come her way, or else she goes to pieces. Such a woman cannot remain faithful to her husband, or to one man.

The spirit of competition is another factor which gives the individual of today quite a bit of difficulty. In order to prove that one is popular many men and their wives act according to the dictates of the crowd. In their gregarious lives they feel it is chic and modern to be in circulation. Nothing can be more damaging in a lifetime partnership than this sort of thinking. Hardly a man or woman who has suffered it can forget the anguish of seeing a wife or husband in the arms of another. The green-horned monster is a persistent devil who rears his ugly head at every opportunity down through the years. Nothing contributes more to depression, insecurity, and mental or emotional unrest than the memory of some real or imagined transgression of a loved one. Such things create doubt and insecurity, which in turn create stress, which in turn becomes anxiety and worse.

Preventive medicine is the cure. Seduction – constant efforts at seduction is that preventive medicine. The man who wants his wife to want him sexually *must* constantly work at it if he is to get what he wants. It is not enough just to be a sexual athlete or to be well endowed physically. One must be a fulltime lover. When this is remembered – and practiced diligently by both sexes – then seduction truly is the spice of life.

THE PROBLEMS of seduction, quite naturally, are too like those of actual lovemaking to be considered or categorized separately. A great deal of the art of seduction *is* in the realm of lovemaking, since seduction is largely a matter of seducing a love partner for the express purpose of making love. To some people, particularly those who feel they are missing something in love and life, it never occurs that their lives would be richer and fuller *if* they devoted a little more time to their love lives. This chapter then, and the subsequent ones, may be of special and particular interest to them for the text is concerned with the 'How' of leading a fuller, richer, and more satisfying love life. The experiences of others are the best teachers – provided, of course, one is willing to learn. Hence, the material that follows is drawn from case histories and other sources to provide the reader with a diverse variety of problems which have been faced – and solved – by others. For simplicity, a question-answer format is generally adopted in the presentation of this case history material. Those questions which appear to concern the great majority of couples have been answered with first person narratives taken from illustrative examples, quoted in part from more than three thousand actual case histories.

My wife feels guilty about sex and refuses to discuss it and our problems. She consents reluctantly to let me make love to her. We have been married two years. She is twenty and has had a very rigid up-bringing. She will not discuss this with our family physician. What can I do?

There is very little you can do, except to be patient and try to give her understanding and love – and to convince her she ought to see a psychologist or physician who can consult with her on a less personal and more professional guidance basis. Very often a young woman of high moral upbringing is fraught with conflicts concerning her love 'duties' to her husband and her own sensual feelings. Study and analysis has shown that a large percentage of young women who have manifested similar restrictive beliefs are usually willing and eager to dispel their guilts when encouraged to do so. An understanding and patient husband can accomplish wonders in this respect *when* he uses the correct seduction and lovemaking technique. Frequently, the moral idea of 'righteousness' is in direct conflict with the individual's sex impulses. When inadequately fulfilled the frustrated sex drive can affect an individual psychologically or emotionally. Each individual problem is different and must be overcome in such a way that the problem is resolved according to the peculiarity and needs of the individual.

At times literature, motion pictures, and the introduction of new acquaintances may work wonders in helping the individual to attain a new 'slant' on life.

A couple with a similar problem resolved their difficulty merely by associating with people from a different social background. The wife, who had been brought up in a convent school, gradually disassociated herself from her girlhood chums, many of whom had erroneous and rather immature ideas about marital relations. She learned, after a few short months, from other young married girls her own age, that life was meant to be enjoyed – not denied or thwarted by religious or moral restriction and superstition. This was effectively brought about when the suffering husband suggested that his wife 'talk sex' with girls and women who were acquaintances of hers at the office where she was employed. A few adroit questions soon opened her eyes and she gradually came to realize that she had been shortchanging herself *and* her husband because of her foolish ideas.

Sometimes when a family physician or someone 'close' to the individual is queried about such matters, help is not received because intimate matters cannot be discussed freely and openly in depth with a 'family friend.' A disinterested person is more apt to give adequate counsel than one who has close emotional ties. For this reason many physicians wisely refer their family and personal friends to other doctors and specialists when advice or counsel is sought. They know that the professional advice of a stranger is often heeded and respected, more so than that given by a friend.

Again, it is important to the harmony of the marital relationship for the husband to understand this. He *must* first overcome his partner's misconceptions and fears before he can effectively teach her to satisfactorily respond to his lovemaking efforts.

Remember, a change of pace always works wonders – and when one broadens one's acquaintanceship with others, the ideas to be garnered and the things to be learned are frequently amazing 'eye openers'. 'Seek and ye shall find.' If youth only *knew* and if only old age *could*. We get too old too soon and smart too late. Learn before it is too late.

One enterprising husband obtained several reels of obscene motion picture film which he showed to his wife. The girl, though shocked at first, admitted that seeing the films changed her entire outlook on life. 'I had no idea people really did those things. Seeing those films was an eye opener to me. I wasn't shocked at what those people were filmed doing – what shocked me – and rudely awakened me – was seeing the women actually enjoying themselves. I just could not believe that women enjoyed sex as much as men did until I saw it with my own eyes.'

24

Frequently, so-called pornography in the form of books, magazines, snapshots and films, is useful in 'opening the eyes' of many individuals who need to learn the truth – even if it is brutally frank. Yes, even pornography has its place in society because it most definitely fills a social need.

What should I do after I've petted my wife and she still fails to respond sexually? She says she wants to be passionate, but she has no feeling in her vaginal area. Our doctor pronounced her normal in every way. She has reached an orgasm several times during the five years of our marriage, but she still cannot be made passionate.

Perhaps the trouble is in *how* you've made preliminary love to your wife. Since she has had sexual gratification infrequently, this does not mean she is incapable of achieving satisfaction whenever it is desired. The fault may be in your technique. Here is how a young married man with a similarly frigid natured wife solved his problem.

'After I had read practically every book I could obtain in which lovemaking techniques were spelled out, I was still unable to arouse Mae. She was willing, but she just couldn't pretend. She told me she loved me and she was glad to satisfy me, but that sex didn't excite her.

'I suppose I started to brood about this, and then begin to feel rejected. That's when I met Patty, an inventory clerk who works at my company. Patty had been married and divorced. She had been around a great deal and she "understood" me. We went to a motel a few times and we hit it off swell. In fact, it was from Patty that I learned *how* to turn a woman on. She was bold and frank and she liked to use coarse language – said it excited her. She really got me all worked up, and I mean she didn't need liquor to do it either. Her secret? She made me feel as if I was the world's greatest lover. She taught me what she liked and what turned her on. After a while it got so that our love-making fell into a routine of sorts. Of course, I broke off the affair with Patty when I saw I was getting into a situation there would be no escape from, and went back to my wife – a sadder and wiser – and more experienced man.

'I used the knowledge I had learned from Patty and before long, my wife, Mae, began to respond – and outperform my former mistress! This is what I used to do and later on, what I began to do to make Mae respond to me . . .

'At first, Mae and I used to neck for awhile. I would caress her breasts and play with her clitoris, but she said my fingers were too rough and it hurt her. She and I used to neck for hours and it never seemed to get her all hot and bothered, though it did fire *me* up.

'I had heard about using your tongue and mouth to make a woman, but hadn't known how until Patty taught me. When I started to kiss my wife's breasts, she tried to push my mouth away and I told her there was nothing to be afraid of. She was reluctant, but she let me. After awhile, her nipples grew rigid under my tongue and I moved my head down over her naked body to kiss her stomach. She tried to fight me away but I told her I loved her and wanted to do what I was doing. She clenched her pillow over her face and finally let me spread her legs open. I kissed her navel and her hips and all around her thighs. This relaxed her a great deal and she soon began to wriggle a little bit. I pressed my mouth to her vulva and found her clitoris with my tongue. I gently titilated her clitoris with my tongue and she began to churn her hips and even began to clutch my head. She was soon ready and we had a right exciting intercourse session after that. We reached orgasm together and it was sublime.

'Later, I tried to question Mae a little, to ask why she hadn't wanted me to kiss her all over, but she was too embarrassed to talk about it. I asked why she had tried to bury her face under the pillow and she again seemed shy and almost ashamed. I told her that the most beautiful sight in the world was the sight of the body of the woman you love. I wanted to watch her face when I kissed her all over because it gave me pleasure to know that I was giving her pleasure. She said she'd try and the next time we made love, she didn't cover her face.

'Before too much longer she was eager for me to titilate her clitoris with my tongue. Though she may be tired or low in spirits, that kind of kissing never fails to arouse her sexually. At first she used to say that it wasn't right to make love like that, but I showed her in at least three different sex books where cunnilingus is practiced by most married couples.

'I found the trick to making her passionate was not in treating her roughly, but in treating her gently and lovingly. Invariably she would get excited and ready for intercourse within a few minutes. Sometimes if I made love to her like that for too long, she'd reach an orgasm while I was tonguing her. She said it wasn't as satisfactory as doing it that way at first, then finishing with regular intercourse, but it nevertheless was enjoyable.'

Frequently, the male may resort to other tactics to whet the female with desire. Massage of the female body will often arouse physical desire, especially if it is done gently and with patience. Many women respond to kisses and caresses on their erogenous zones such as the neck, ear, breast, buttocks, backs of the knees, small of the back, hips, thighs and stomach. It has been found that a great number of women are particularly more sensitive in areas outside the pubic region.

Skillful titilation of the clitoris with finger or tongue will usually succeed when all else fails. The woman who is slow to respond erotically will usually become passionate when she is caressed lovingly and patiently. Woman's nature is such that she must feel secure in what she is doing in order to enjoy the sex act to the utmost. The man who takes this into consideration, then makes love in a patient and unhurried fashion, succeeds.

I am quite a bit taller and heavier than my wife and she is fearful of having intercourse with me because she admits that I sometimes hurt her when I'm on top facing her. What must I do to help her overcome this fear? She says that if she wasn't so afraid that I might hurt her when I get carried away in the throes of passion, she might enjoy sex relations with me more and would like to have them more often than twice or three times weekly. What can I do?

Twenty-seven year old Edmund F., a former football star weighing two hundred-forty pounds and who is six-feet five has this to say when telling a physician how he overcame the same fear which had been expressed by his five-foot tall wife, Aggie.

'After we had been married several months Aggie finally confessed the reason why she had been so reluctant to let me make love to her: she was scared that I'd hurt her. I went to a doctor and told him my problem. He gave me a complete physical examination. He told me my wife ought not have anything to fear because we didn't have to make love in the traditional way facing each other with the man on top. He suggested that we try some variations, preferably with the wife on top.

'I told Aggie this and she felt abashed, embarrassed or whatever because she had always thought doing it any way other than the woman on the bottom was lewd. When she couldn't overcome this fear despite what I said, I insisted that she see a doctor who would set her straight. Now Aggie is a regular sort of girl with plenty on the ball – so she thought, *until* the doctor consulted with her and gave her the scoop. He found out something I hadn't been able to learn: that Aggie had some very foolish and backward ideas about sex. For one thing she thought that sex relations should only be enjoyed for a few minutes at a time and that it was wrong and unhealthy to prolong love-making. The doctor corrected her misconceptions and later we talked over what had been discussed and what she had learned. We did better than just talk things over –

we tried them out.

'Aggie and I went to bed and I kissed and fondled her, face down on top of me. She was very embarrassed, so I covered us with a sheet and that seemed to make her feel more at ease. I played with her until I felt that her vagina was moist enough and ready, then I held her by the hips and pressed up into her. She was very afraid and cautious, but when she saw that I was not hurting her and was able to control my movements better, she let herself go. I told her I loved her and I could kiss her breasts and she liked that. It was the first time I had ever been able to lick her nipples while we were having sex relations. On top, I could never seem to bend myself down far enough to kiss her breasts at the same time.

'Before long she began to feel more secure and she let herself go. She kept asking me if I felt that she was being brazen, and of course I assured her that she wasn't. She felt better about this and had a terrific orgasm. I continued to make love to her afterwards and she had a second orgasm, much to her surprise.

'We tried many other positions and found that it was very good in a chair with her sitting on my penis, facing me. That way I could hold her buttocks and regulate her movements and my own. Soon we were doing it backwards, too – with she kneeling in a crouch, her buttocks jutting up toward the edge of the bed. I could enter her vagina from the rear and also play with her clitoris with my fingers as I was loving her. We sometimes made love face to face on our sides, but the best position of all was with Aggie on top. She has learned that it excites me a great deal to see her like that and she enjoys the act very much now because she has learned to prolong it and let herself go. Occasionally, when I mount her in the man-above position, she still freezes up somewhat, but she isn't as afraid of me as she used to be. Whenever we do it that way, I try to keep my weight off her by supporting my body on my arms. However, due to our difference in physical size, the woman-above position is ideal for us.'

29

I require sex relations more than my husband does. Sometimes I am able to arouse his desire by fondling his genitals, but that doesn't seem to give him an erection as frequently as I'd like. If I kiss and take his penis in my mouth [which is something I have a strong urge to do] will this work? And will he think bad things about me if I do that?

The following excerpt from a typical case history provides the answer:

'My husband loves me and enjoys sexual intercourse, but he never took the initiative when we were first married. He always waited for me to make the first overtures sexually and he obliged and always satisfied me. But lately, because he has been under a great deal of mental strain because of his job, he seems to be totally uninterested in sex, though he doesn't complain about it when I ask him.

'I suppose I began to feel unwanted or unloved or rejected or something like that because I felt a stronger and stronger urge to have sex with him. I think about sex a great deal and I would often be ready, willing and anxious to make love the moment he entered the door when he came home after work of an evening. But as time went by he began to lose interest and several times, after I had fondled his organ for a long time, he failed to get an erection.

'The other night, after I had gone without sex for nearly a week, I decided to hell with convention and everything else and I would do what I felt the urge to do. He got into bed and was fast asleep the second his head hit the pillow. I took off my nightgown, then I pulled off his pajama trousers. He didn't budge.

'I hugged and kissed him and he still did not move. I began to kiss his chest and then his stomach, but that didn't awaken him either. All it did was make me hotter and hotter. I got this strong urge to fondle and caress his penis. I did and I was soon trembling, I was that passionate. I kissed it and he moaned and stirred a little, but he didn't protest and didn't try to push my head away. I then took the head of his penis in my mouth and sucked it gently, rolling my tongue around the glans. He started to get rigid and he responded by taking my head in his hands and caressing my hair. I continued moving my head and working my tongue all around. Soon he had a rigid, throbbing erection and he was wide awake. He pushed me up and then mounted me. We made love vigorously and when it was over, fell asleep in each other's arms.

'Later, when we discussed it, he said he had liked what I had done to him practicing fellatio – and had always wanted it, but was reluctant to ask me to do it to him that way because he was afraid I would find it distasteful. Quite the contrary, I enjoy it and it gives me great pleasure to see him enjoy it so much. Sometimes I let him reach a climax in my mouth and when he does that he usually moves around to put his head between my legs and kisses my clitoris and vulva so we can have an orgasm at the same time.

'Now whenever he is tired and doesn't take the initiative, I take his penis in my mouth and love it and tease it until it is stiff and hard. That does things to him that are simply unbelievable. We are able to have vigorous sexual relations when we seduce each other that way. It seems to awaken him better than any other technique I know.'

'Frankly, if my husband would have thought badly of me for being so forward and doing that to him, I would have been sure he didn't love me. As it was, I was rapidly reaching that point in married life when I couldn't stand being frustrated any longer, and if he would not have responded to me, I think I would have taken a lover or asked for a divorce.'

My husband is gentle and loving and considerate of me. He seduces me after much necking and petting, but when he is ready to have intercourse, either he loses his erection or he ejaculates prematurely. What shall I do?

Obviously, the husband is still unskilled and inept in the art of seduction and lovemaking. He has not learned the secrets of mastering one's self-control enough to prolong the sex act sufficiently for mutual enjoyment. When this happens, it is frequently the wife who must take steps to alleviate the situation. Here is how twenty-nine year old Alice D., a wife and mother of three small children corrected her husband's inadequacy. Alice D. relates:

'Steve is one of those guys who think they know it all, but who really doesn't know as much as he'd like others to think. And so it was with our love life until I just couldn't stand his bungling another minute. After seven years of reasonably happy married life [except for our sex relations] Stevie still hadn't learned how to stay erect long enough to satisfy me also. He would neck and caress me and by the time I was steaming hot and my vagina was bathed in moisture, he would get on top of me, then ejaculate immediately. Sometimes he would last maybe a few seconds, but most of the time he would come before he had fully penetrated me. Then he would roll over and go to sleep and leave me panting. More than once I put myself to sleep only after I masturbated myself.

'I asked my doctor about this and he suggested that perhaps I ought to give him more sex than I had been accustomed to so that he might be less excited when it came time for us to make love. He said that frequently men would ejaculate prematurely because they are too excited and cannot control themselves. He said that sometimes a mild alcoholic drink or a tranquilizer might calm them down, but he didn't know and he asked if I would bring Steve round to see him.

'Well, Steve just wouldn't hear of it. He was angry at me for even suggesting such a thing. I argued with him and told him how unfairly he'd been treating me. Well, he was quite surprised and even shocked because he hadn't known, or thought about it. We had never discussed it before, strangely enough. This was primarily what was wrong. We went to bed and made up our minds to overcome his problem no matter what. But, as soon as he put his penis against my vulva, before he could penetrate, he ejaculated again. I was furious, but I didn't let on. I kept kissing him and fondling his organ and before too much longer he was erect again. I might add that this was the first time since we'd been on our honeymoon that he had had two erections the same evening. I then encouraged him and we had a glorious intercourse. It lasted for almost an hour before we both – for the first time since we'd married – reached a climax at the same time.

'After that I would always make certain that we had relations every night and sometimes in the morning too, in order that he grow accustomed to having intercourse. As time went by, he no longer had a quick ejaculation. He got so he was able to prolong his erection for an hour or more – with my help and encouragement, of course. And of course, we enjoy ourselves immensely.

'Actually, my hubby's trouble was due to the fact that neither of us communicated – we had failed to tell each other what was on our minds. When we had done this, Steve was more than willing to satisfy me. We have a great time in bed together now. I no longer feel frustrated and out of sorts. He has also responded by being more alert and less tired all the time. Now when he boasts of his sexual prowess, I wink at him knowingly.

My wife performs fellatio on me and when she does she insists that I do cunnilingus on her. Is this harmful?

A consensus by professionals is that neither fellatio nor cunnilingus is harmful, provided it is practiced with moderation and does not become the sole method of sexual gratification. Both fellatio and cunnilingus, when practiced by couples who are dear to one another, are seduction or lovemaking *preliminaries*, and should be indulged only to derive the maximum satisfaction therefrom, when followed by sexual intercourse. Such mouth-genital

33

contact has been practiced by man since time immemorial and there is no doubt will continue to be practiced without harm to man or woman. With some individuals, intensity of sexual feeling and desire is increased greatly when oral stimulus is used. The intimacy between couples who are in love knows no restrictions, taboos, nor limitations. Only when the act is offensive to either of the parties should it be avoided.

How can I tempt my husband to make love to me when I desire him, yet am unable to boldly make overtures to him?

Timid twenty-one year old Millie K. made this statement to a psychologist by whom she was being counseled. It is apropros of this quite common problem and it provides an adequate answer.

'I did as you suggested, Doctor, and you know, it worked! Davy just wouldn't take the initiative because he respects me so much and because he's afraid of I don't know what – until I tried seducing him by wearing sexy clothes. He is passionate and so am I, so we have no problem on that score. But when it comes right down to talking about it matter-of-factly, he turns red as a beet and changes the subject. His embarrassment has made me equally as self conscious about having sexual intercourse more frequently than one or two times a week. I would like it every night and since I've been doing what you suggested, we have had relations every night. Davy can't resist me now.

'Last week, I wore a filmy transparent negligée in the kitchen as I washed the dishes. He started hugging me while he dried the dishes and we never did get finished doing those dishes that night. The next night, after supper, I took a shower and came downstairs to watch TV with Davy, wearing only a terrycloth wrapper. I let it open so my breasts and thighs were exposed and again he couldn't resist. We made love on the rug in the living room that night.

'I now have learned that whenever I want him to make love to me, all I have to do is wear something enticing or seductive that reveals and conceals and mystifies. This excites him and he goes after me like a male animal. I knew about such things, but I never knew they really worked. Lately, I've been getting bolder, too – and so has Davy. We've overcome some of our former embarrassment and who knows, maybe someday we'll both be cured – but I like it this way now.'

What am I to think when my wife lets me kiss and pet her and then refuses to let me have intercourse with her? Is she merely torturing me or am I that incapable of arousing sexual desire in her?

There are many and various reasons why a woman will reject her husband moments before she is about to surrender sexually. Some women freely admit that they are abhorred by the crude manner of approach used by their mates. Others admit that they are in the mood to have sexual intercourse, but the mannerisms or actions of their mates repulse them and kill their desire.

The rejection at the last minute is certainly frustration personified for either or both parties; but this need not be the rule rather than the exception when certain common-sense precautions are taken.

Foul breath and unpleasant body odors can do more toward alienating affections than most people care to admit. When a man has a garlic-laden breath or when a woman has an unpleasant odor about her body, nothing can be more disconcerting to the sexually aroused individual than this. Care about hygiene and bodily cleanliness is a must. If one has indulged in alcohol or onion-flavored dishes, the precaution of using mouthwashes or breath sweeteners is not unwise.

Some men alienate their wive's sexual attraction for them by conscious or unconscious mannerisms which are frequently obnoxious and distasteful. For example, many men patiently make love to their wives, taking care to arouse them sexually, then, when the need for continued gentleness is required, they cease being loving and act like overgrown boys. Instead of being gentle and patient, they become impatient and rough, often manhandling their wives like brutes taking a rape victim. They approach them roughly and without gentility and by such actions, thwart any response they might have otherwise have enjoyed.

The great lover many men fancy themselves to be is indeed a misconception – they are too foolish to realize that their behaviour and uncouth attitudes are repugnant to the women they are trying to seduce into having relations with them.

As one woman so aptly stated: 'Won't men ever learn? They wine us and dine us and treat us like royalty, but the moment before we are willing to give in to them sexually, they stop treating us like queens and instead treat us like common street whores. If there's one thing I can't stand, that's a man who treats me like he loves me one minute, then tells me to take off my pants and lay down for him the next minute. Where is their tact, their finesse?'

Enough said?

We've heard a great deal about french kissing, soul kissing, and titilation of the erogenous zones with the tongue, but no one has ever thoroughly explained any of this to us. Will you kindly expound for my wife and I?

The first pleasures of man begin in infancy when he instinctively derives pleasure, comfort, and satisfaction from sucking. The mouth, lips and tongue are distinctive erogenous zones of the human anatomy which are, in and of themselves, quite capable of stimulating the body sexually when in contact with a love partner. There is a strong unconscious wish to bite or suckle the body of a loved one in all of us. Some individuals derive great pleasure from drawing upon the mouth of another; others, from plunging the tongue into the mouth of another. When such sensitive zones are in close contact, either by the joining of mouths or mingling of tongues, the senses are naturally excited and other areas of the human body become susceptible to stimuli.

'French kissing' or soul kissing is more or less the use of the tongue during the kiss. The term 'French kissing' is sometimes erroneously used to mean the 'French way' which describes the act of cunnilingus or fellatio. So long as the practice of tongue kissing is not offensive to either party, such is said to be perfectly permissible a practice.

The use of the lips, nose, ear, throat, and other body areas for titilation of another is commonly in practice throughout the civilised world of today. Very often the man who kisses the throat or breast of his loved one finds himself becoming highly excited by the very intimacy of his caresses. The same holds true of the female who licks or kisses the erogenous zones of the male.

The erogenous zones on the body vary from individual to individual, but most people are aroused sexually when the same parts are caressed or kissed. Most women can be aroused sexually when their breasts are kissed and the nipples are fondled or gently sucked. Exciting the erogenous zones is a simple matter. One woman may become highly aroused when kissed on the back of the neck; another may only become aroused when kissed on the ear, the upper lip, the stomach, the insides of her thighs, or even on the clitoris.

Rapid movements of the tongue across the sensitive nerve endings of one's erogenous zone are both pleasurable and capable of arousal when expertly done. Caresses which range from gentle love bites on the hip, shoulder, knee, thigh, neck, ear, etc. to "butterfly" kisses which are barely more than light caresses with the eyelashes or body hair are equally exciting to most individuals. The Eskimos derive pleasure from nose rubbing, for instance. In some individuals the nostrils are highly erogenous areas and may be extremely sensitive to titilation. In others, the upper or lower lip may be highly susceptible to stimulation, especially by gentle licking or the brushing of lips. Still others find that the sucking of the loved one's flesh on the shoulder, thigh or buttock is enough to induce fiery passion within moments.

The art of kissing is one that requires practice and, of course, experimentation. It most certainly cannot be learned from a book.

Is it possible to arouse my wife sexually just by holding my erect penis against her body? I would like to try this, but I'm afraid she'll think I'm lewd.

The direct answer to this question is, of course, yes. It is possible to arouse a woman sexually by touching the penis against her body, particularly her erogenous zones. Also, it is possible to disgust her, or repulse her when this is done crudely and without preliminary lovemaking.

When a couple are in bed together, embracing, their nude bodies at close proximity there is hardly a woman alive who will believe her lover to be lewd if he touches her with his erect penis. Contrarily, such a gesture is expected, for when it is done in a natural manner and used as a means of caressing and exciting, it cannot be construed as being an 'obscene' act. In fact, it is both highly exciting and pleasurable to the female. When making such an attempt, it is wise to wait until the proper moment when the female's passions have been aroused sufficiently to obtain a favorable response. The uncouth man who unzips, and waggles his penis promiscuously is doing more to defeat his purpose than he is to encourage feminine interest in him. Only on rare instances have women been known to respond favorably to a man who turns to exhibitionism in order to entice them. There are many instances when long-married couples have refrained from exposing their bodies to each other for fear of offending. Many psychologists and psychiatrists have stated that not infrequently they have clients and patients who have never seen the genitals of their mates!

Everything depends upon the individuals in their particular circumstances as to what they do and how they may be expected to react to sex stimuli. To some, the fondling of the loved one's genitals is an unpleasant thing – to others, it is the height of ecstasy and the very epitome of love expression.

I had had intercourse with numerous women before I married for the first time. My wife is inexperienced, though she was not a virgin at the time we were married. We have been married for a year now and there are some things I want to teach her about how to have intercourse and all, but I'm afraid that if I attempt to teach her, she'll be upset because I learned those things from having done them with other girls. How do I overcome this?

The case history of a former actor, Eric J., will best answer this query. Eric had this to say to his psychiatrist a few months after his therapy had ended:

'Joanne was young and innocent and rather in awe of me, I must confess – which was why I was that considerate and gentle with her all the time. Little did I know at the time we were married that she had been particularly fascinated by me because I had been such a ladies' man before I settled down with her. I found out much later that Joanne had had this affair with a guy from her home town. He was a bungler and his attempts to have intercourse with her were unpleasant, painful, and frustrating to her. Joanne was – and still is – quite a sexy girl. She wanted me to teach her all I knew because she wanted to have sex with me in every way possible; but, she was reluctant to speak up because she was afraid I'd lose respect for her if I knew.

'I was also afraid to teach her what I had learned because I was afraid she'd be disillusioned about me. She's a sweet, demure, sensitive girl and I suppose I always was afraid of hurting or shocking her – which was why, I guess, I broke her in gradually and refused to teach her.

'One day when we had an argument it all came out. She screamed at me and accused me of being a phoney – that I had never been the "lover" everyone claimed I was – that I couldn't satisfy her!

'Which was why I began to think that perhaps I needed psychiatric help, Doctor. I thought that maybe something *was* wrong with me. Now I know differently. I was, of course, sexually immature, but I got over that in due time, thanks to your help and therapy. However, what I failed to realize was that I had some secret guilt feelings about my sexual excesses before marriage. I had believed those old wives' tales about too much sex before marriage weakening the semen and causing deformity in children. I worried about this and I guess that was the reason I became impotent with my wife. My fear of teaching her was overcome and I was able to perform adequately and was like my old self again.

'I learned that Joanne was quite pleased to have married me and that she enjoyed hearing about how much "better" she was in bed than any other woman I'd had before her. Contrary to my fears, she was eager to learn. She wanted to outperform other women I'd had. She had wanted to marry an "experienced" man so she could learn all there was to know. When I realized this, we talked things over in intimate detail. Our relations improved at once. Two things cured me: one, overcoming the erroneous belief that my children would be deformed because of my so called premarital sexual excesses; and two, baring my soul to my wife who in turned shared her confidences. This has brought us closer together than ever and we are grateful that we've reached this new plateau of understanding.'

The techniques of seduction and lovemaking are indeed

many and varied. What is pleasurable and gratifying to one couple may not be likewise to another couple. All that matters in the sexual union is that the tastes and preferences of the individual are agreeable to the partner – therefore, 'no holds barred' lovemaking techniques *are* acceptable when both partners condone and enjoy them. No such thing as obscenity or 'deviation' occurs in a union in which both partners are gratified by their intimacies. According to the needs, both emotional, psychological, and physical, of the individual partners, 'everything goes' when the art of seduction and lovemaking takes place. This is the secret of finding new freedom and pleasure in the sexual life. When erroneous guilts, fears, and misconceptions are brought out in the open, the emotional barriers to free expression through love are lowered and the individual may freely enjoy life as it was meant to be enjoyed – in the arms of a loved one.

On Seducing A Bride

SOCIETY has imposed a double standard of behavior upon the single man and woman. It is 'acceptable' for the male to have numerous affairs, but *not* acceptable for the female to do likewise. Although the emancipation of the woman has been more complete during recent decades, it still remains 'indecent' of her to 'love them and leave them' as does the male. Man still enjoys more sexual freedom than woman. He may have brief sexual encounters and prolonged affairs without being condemned by society. On the other hand, the girl who does the same is looked upon with disdain. In most cases she is expected to be a virgin when she is married. Then she is expected to fulfill her husband's needs in every way without any prior experience. Her sexual urges are considered by society to be nonexistent prior to her wedding night at which magical time she is supposed to throw off the Victorian chastity belt for the first time.

Does this make sense? Of course not.

Society fails to recognize that times have changed. The advent of modern hygienic devices and 'the pill' have made it easy for the female to consort as freely as the male. But when she does submit to her lover prior to marriage what happens? Is her fiancé disappointed? Is he frightened off? Does he back out of the marriage? Is he one of those who feel that now, since he has deflowered his bride to be, why bother to marry her?

Strangely, many men who would otherwise *not* have married the women they married, did marry because their fiancées *were* virgins on the wedding day. This remains one of the major reasons why so many young men are lured into marriage for the first time. They have 'sown their wild oats' and now they are ready to settle down. They have found 'the girl of their dreams' and they have fallen in love with her – yet, they have never slept with her. They have known many others, but not their brides intimately. Are they entering a platonic love affair which is to remain so for the rest of their lives? Or are they really obsessed with the idea that the bride is a virgin? And why are they so certain that this marriage – to a woman of untested sexual capacity or ability – is *the* right one?

The major reason why so many first marriages end in disappointment and failure in the divorce courts is because the couples do not really know each other – and have not known each other sufficiently well prior to getting married. Nothing is truer than that old maxim: 'You never know someone until you've slept and lived with him or her'.

How is it possible then to determine whether a girl will be a good wife if the young man courting her never sees her as she really is? Moreover, how is he to know if she is compatible if he has never had sexual relations with her? If the man is of a rather healthy physical makeup, how can he expect a frail, diminutive young lady of rather sedentary habits to keep up with him socially, physically and sexually? If the man has been accustomed to vigorous and frequent sexual affairs, how can he be expected to remain faithful to his wife who remains passive and does not 'enjoy' physical relations with her husband? How long will he remain true to a woman who frustrates him night after night? How patient will he be when he must teach his bride the nuances of lovemaking? He has spent his boyhood and young adulthood in sexual adventure and experimentation – his bride has been uninitiated until their wedding day. How *can* she be expected to match him when she is inexperienced and virginal?

When frustration has begun to dull the glitter of excitement of young marriage, the bride announces she is pregnant. Whether this is deliberate to keep the errant husband from leaving the household, or if this is unconsciously motivated, cannot be determined. The point is, the couple remain married to each other and perhaps – for the sake of the child and later children – they learn to live with each other.

This is not to say that all marriages are unhappy or unsatisfactory. The contrary is true.

We have mentioned the foregoing briefly to prepare the reader for what is to follow. We have shown that sexuality is oftentimes the main reason why men and women marry. Companionship, social enjoyment and security are important too, but with youthful, healthy persons the biological urge is the dominant factor that attracts young people.

When one is stirred with sexual cravings reason is often distorted. An upright young man who is dating a young lady 'falls madly in love' with her and soon proposes. His relatives and friends tell him the girl is 'wrong' for him. They argue with him endlessly, showing him her faults; how unsuitable she is, etc. But all to no avail. His love for her is truly blind. She has accepted him and his lust for her must be sated no matter what. He is overwrought with anxiety. In this state he cannot think clearly. He pictures life with his lady love as being sublime with a fairy tale ending. He cannot see her as she really is. He is blind to her faults. He cannot visualize how her habits may grate on his nerves; how her personality may conflict with his own. Others can see the disparity, but he is blind. Why? Because his frustrated sex drive has been fixated upon her. He has wearied of finding sexual satisfaction whenever and wherever he could find it. Now he wants to settle down to an idyllic existence. He wants a wife with whom he can indulge his sexual fancies. He wants a companion who will help him to escape from a humdrum existence. He is tired of the hurt of being rejected by women he has dated; he has wearied of the never ending hunt for sexual relief; and the love of his

44

life promises to take him 'away' to a never-never land where all will be sweetness and light.

If she is a virtuous woman then he considers himself very fortunate.

Though he wants her and the weeks or months before the wedding date place the magical time of sexual release and bliss in the distant future, she still keep him at arms length. Why?

Is she afraid he will be disappointed and will break off the engagement? Probably. Is she afraid for other reasons? Probably. She cannot understand man's constant drive to seduce woman. Even at her tender age and her naïvely virginal period in life she knows that man must be held at bay. Perhaps she has spent many amorous hours fighting off those who wanted to take her virginity from her. Perhaps she has grown accustomed to this feeling of power over men and perhaps she enjoys it to the extent that she intends to keep her husband at bay too.

She agrees to marry because she is 'in love'. But how often is that state of being 'in love' false? How often does she agree to marry because she wants to live her own life and escape from a humdrum existence, of being dominated by parents, of being frustrated in other ways? How often does she consent to marriage because she has been 'swept off her feet' with a whirlwind courtship? How often does she promise to marry when she knows intellectually that the man is not suited to her; but she wants to marry him anyway to prove that she is something special to her friends who are not being 'rushed' by eligible young men?

We could go on and on. But such discussion is unnecessary. The reader is aware of the many and various reasons why people marry. When the emotions bar the intellect from making sound decisions, look out – trouble is in the offing. When ardor cools, the volcano explodes.

What then is the solution? How does a young man or lady determine what is right? There is only one answer. Experience. Experience is the best – and often, the *only* teacher. How then does one go about gaining experience?

45

By practicing the art of seduction.

Let's consider a typical problem. A young lady to whom a certain young man is engaged is supposed to have a volatile temper. The young man has been warned that he could never put up with a shrewish temper, complete with childish tantrums, as that displayed by his bride-to-be. How then, can he find out for himself when she is on her best behavior whenever he sees her?

Simple – seduce her into getting angry. Goad her into losing her temper. Then will be the acid test.

The young man took the advice, and sure enough he, saw the ugly vehemence of his short-tempered fiancée. He realized that he could not live with that behavior. The question next to be considered was whether he can change her. The answer obviously is no. He cannot undo a behavior pattern or characteristic which was twenty years in the making.

Next question – how can he break off the engagement when he is sure, that despite her ugly temper, he is in love with her?

Breaking off the engagement is one thing – *preparing* himself for it is another. Apparently he was possessed with the idea of making love to her. Whether or not this has been sublimated is questionable. What matters is that he wanted her physically and his libido has been stirred to such heights that he will have no other woman until he has her.

The truth, then, is the only way out.

He confronted her straightforwardly. 'Darling, for some time I've been hearing about your terrible temper. I love you despite it, I want you to know – but I'm not sure of one thing. I'm not sure if I really am in love with you or if my attraction toward you is purely physical.'

The girl reacted by slapping him in the face.

The engagement ended and the young man was spared an unhappy relationship. His former fiancée married another soon afterward and that marriage ended in divorce.

When a couple suspects that their attraction for each

46

other is largely physical, how can they possible determine if they are truly 'in love' and if they are suited to each other? How can they discover the truth when their emotions are so intertwined with unrequited sexual desires? In the state many engaged couples find themselves emotionally, how can they differentiate physical desire from 'love' before it is too late and they take their marriage vows?

A prominent psychologist advised a young man, who had been seeking his counsel on just such a problem, to make an 'inventory' of his fiancée's faults and attributes. 'Take plenty of time,' he said, 'to enumerate everything you can think of that's good and bad about her. Then try to separate the things about her which you feel have attracted you to her. Be honest with yourself. Ask yourself if your emotional attachment toward her is heavily sexual – if you have near-masturbatory fantasies about her – if she represents a sex-love object to you which has heretofore been unobtainable. Finally, ask yourself if you would marry her *if* she permitted you to make love to her – *if* she were not a virgin.'

The young man spent several days making a list of his fiancée's good and bad points. He was as objective as he could be. When he arrived at the psychologist's office for his next appointment, he had this to say:

'I've known Karen for ten months and you know, this is the first time I actually sat down and tallied up the facts. She can't cook. She isn't thrifty. She's vain as a peacock. She is always concerned about impressing her girls friends and lording it over them. She's temperamental and high-strung. And in the cold light of day I can see no reason, other than sexual, to love her. Frankly doctor, I have been impressed with her femininity and beauty and I do want her sexually – but, aside from the sex part there is nothing else about her that is compatible with me. If she isn't as sexy as she lets on, I'm afraid our marriage will be a bust.'

The young man soon accepted the truth of the situation. He was obsessed with the idea that his fiancée was attractive and he had a strong physical desire for her. Her attractiveness and the fact that she was a 'good catch' impressed him more than anything else about her. He was determined to possess her sexually no matter what. Eventually he admitted to himself that he would *not* think of marrying her if she were not a virgin. He also admitted that this was an unrealistic viewpoint – a foolish fixation. He broke off the engagement and has not regretted it.

There are other ways and means to clear the vision of those blinded by love. Since marriage is intended to be a life-long parternship it should be entered into intelligently. Engagements should be made with the intellect, not the emotions. When a man and a woman are free of sexual frustrations they are capable of making more sensible or rational decisions about marriage. The following case history illustrates this.

Case No. 581
Richard S. Age 28
The subject visited a psychiatrist because he was unsure of himself and felt 'nervous and upset' about a forthcoming marriage, his first. He was lacking in confidence and unsure of his love for the girl he was engaged to. He sought psychiatric advice because he was becoming increasingly apprehensive and insecure. Acute indigestion and extreme anxiety had made him uncomfortable and restless. He was unable to sleep. He wanted to know why.

After five weeks of analysis he finally learned the answers for himself. The following is a transcript of a discussion which took place on his last and final visit to the therapist.

'Yes, Doctor, I think I see the point. I've always been a worry wart and I suppose I instinctively knew that something was not right about my engagement to Doris but I just couldn't face up to it or put my finger on it. Until now, that is.

'I came to you five weeks ago because I felt depressed and nervous. The indigestion and insomnia were due to worry, I knew. I also knew that I was worried about taking the big step with Doris. In fact, this was making me sick, worrying. Now that I've resolved some things in my own mind I believe I can unwind and relax.

'I told Doris last week after my visit here to you, Doctor, that I was seeing a psychiatrist. I told her what was bothering me and that I was deeply concerned to the point of utter nervousness. I confessed to her that I had been having sexual relations with other girls on an average of two or more times a week ever since I was seventeen. I stopped having sexual intercourse with other girls six months ago when we were first engaged. I never tried to have sex relations with her because I respected and loved her and I wanted to be true to her as she had promised she would be true to me too.

'She told me she admired and loved me for being faithful to her and that was as it should be. She said she had hoped I would continue being faithful to her until we get married two months from now.

'I told her that that was just the trouble. I had this strong sexual feeling toward her and I just couldn't think straight because of it. Everything about her is terrific, but she doesn't allow me to get intimate, or even to pet with her. In fact, she was one of the few girls I've known in my lifetime who refused to let me pet her. So, I began to wonder if maybe I was just obsessed with the idea of marrying her just to have her sexually. I told her this and she laughed. She kissed me and said that she understood and that I was just growing nervous as the time for our wedding approached.

'I told her that I wasn't nervous about that. Instead I was worried if I really cared enough to marry her if the sex part wasn't so important to me. She was upset when I told her that, but she said she understood. Then she surprised me by asking if I wanted to go to bed with her before our wedding night.

'Naturally, I said yes. I told her that since we were already engaged what difference did it make? Besides, if we were not compatible sexually, would that make a difference to both of us? I meant that I was worried if we didn't hit it off well sexually; would we get along okay in other things like the everyday business of living?

'She thought about it and said that we owed it to ourselves to be sure before we married. About each other, that is. She said that she didn't know I was sick worrying about it, and she was glad I had been honest with her. She didn't want me to be sick – and she didn't want me to go to any other girl for sexual relief. She said she loves me and she'd do anything to make me happy. So, we went away together last weekend. It was the first time for us. We went to a resort and checked into a nice hotel. There was nothing sordid about it. She and I slept together for the first time. It was just like being on a preview of a honeymoon. She was pretty ignorant about what to do so I taught her. She was willing to learn and eager to please. She had satisfied me sexually and I had satisfied her, too. She was glad and so was I. I told her that I was sure about her and she was pleased. Since then I've been secure in my thinking and I am not bothered with indigestion or insomnia.'

Richard seduced his bride-to-be prior to their wedding because he was honest with her. She had a choice to make and she was later glad she had made it. She was intelligent enough to realize that Richard *was* distraught and upset because he had been faithful to her and had stopped having relations with other girls. His sexual abstinence was causing his distress. She knew that they were well suited to each other and that the problem of sex was not going to come between them if she could help it. Moreover, she later admitted to Richard, she also had been concerned if his interest in her was largely of a sexual nature. She was satisfied that it wasn't – other things in life mattered too.

The moral of this case history is evident: the direct

approach of the truth is usually the best way to seduce a woman. Doris saw that Richard was distressed enough to see a psychiatrist. She was alarmed because she knew she was partly to blame. She knew he was telling her the truth because he stated it without embellishment. Moreover, she wanted him as badly as he wanted her. She felt the need to show him that he was important to her and that she wanted to please him and share the happiness of love with him.

If Richard had not been truthful with Doris, if he had not told her how upset he had been getting, Doris would not have consented to surrender herself before their wedding day. He did not resort to subterfuge. He merely told the truth and that was all that was needed to seduce Doris.

According to many published works on the subject, a large percentage of brides *do* surrender to their fiancés before their wedding nights. Of those who have been married previously, better than eighty percent have sexual relations prior to marriage. Frequently, many casual sexual affairs bud into serious love affairs that lead to marriage. The pleasure of sexual harmony is just one facet of happiness in life. Compatibility is another. Honor and respect are others. Habit is another. And finally, the security of love – total love – is the crowning joy. Deep, long-lasting mature love between a man and a woman is the most satisfying relationship man and woman can enjoy.

When a couple is in love it is the *non*material things which matter most. When a husband takes the time and the trouble to make a game of seducing his bride, the resulting satisfaction knows no measure of capacity. Joy and sensation is heightened to the very limits of ecstasy. Delight with one another is charged to its maximum. The husband who properly seduces his bride, prospers in more ways than one. The groom who foolishly does not practice the art of seduction impoverishes his marriage. The bride who feels cherished and loved responds with equanimity and her reaction heightens the excitement of togetherness

51

and intimacy. When man is stripped naked of all his possessions, yet still has his bride at his side, he continues to remain rich as long as he is free to be seduced and be the seducer. No matter how discouraged or defeated man can be, nothing exalts his spirit more than the love of one dear to him; and nothing exhilarates him more, or inspires him on, than the wife of his youth whose arms and lips and caresses inflame him with desire. Seduction is just that – the creation of desire, the stimulation of sexual appetite. No matter how sublimated the sex urge may be, the seduction of one person who loves another overcomes that sublimation.

Case No. 717
June B. Age 22
Subject was seen by the marriage counselor at the urging of her newlywed husband. She appeared tense and reluctant to discuss her problem which had already been explained to the counselor by the husband. She was shy and inhibited and surprisingly naïve for a girl who just had been graduated from college. After several visits she overcame her initial timidity and spoke freely of her problem . . .

'I've tried very hard to be a good wife to Earl these past few months of our marriage, but I just do not understand what he expects of me. He says I'm as unresponsive and as sexy as a marble statue in a museum. I suppose I am, and I don't know what to do about it.

'He takes his time making love to me, kissing me and caressing me when we go to bed, but I just don't feel anything. I do love him and I do so want to please him, but he doesn't believe me. I just don't feel anything. Do you suppose I'm frigid?

[The results of a medical examination revealed that June was normal in all respects and there was no physical reason to suspect that she was frigid.]

The marriage counselor, a prominent female Ph.D. from

California went into intimate detail during the interview that followed. Here is a transcript of that discussion:

Doctor: Explain what you mean by frigidity.
June: Well, it's being cold and not feeling anything. I don't get any pleasure out of the sex act.
Doctor: Is it painful?
June: No.
Doctor: Have you ever experienced sexual pleasure? Have you ever had an orgasm?
June: Yes. Before we were married. We used to park sometimes and neck. Earl would play with my breasts and sometimes he put his hand under my dress. He rubbed my clitoris with his fingers and I got an orgasm many times. We were having sex relations for a long time before we were married.
Doctor: Did you feel guilty about having sexual intercourse before you were married?
June: Yes. I suppose I did. Earl laughed at me, but I didn't see the humor of it. I was brought up properly. I felt that having intercourse before marriage was not right.
Doctor: Tell me about your wedding. Was it a formal affair in a church?
June: Oh yes. It was very lovely. I had an exquisite gown for the occasion. Earl wore tails. It was the realization of my dreams. It was positively the most marvelous day of my life – all my friends were there – my parents – me in that white bridal gown – everything was perfect – except that I didn't feel pure like a virgin bride. I couldn't look my mother or my sisters in the face. I felt guilty. I wished Earl wouldn't have insisted.
Doctor: Are you punishing yourself now because you believe you've transgressed with Earl before your wedding night?
June: I never thought about it like that, but now that you mention it, do you suppose that's *why* I can't let myself go now?
Doctor: What do you think?

June: Gosh, I don't know for sure. I'm confused.

Doctor: Did you want Earl to have relations with you when you consented to submit before your wedding?

June: I suppose it would be dishonest of me to say no. Yes, I let him seduce me. I wanted him. I suppose I might have been able to stop him. Yes, I let him seduce me.

Doctor: Why?

June: I'm not sure, really. We were necking at home. My folks were away at the time. I was excited and very passionate. He had brought me up to the point of orgasm several times. Then he undressed me. He undressed too. I was very excited when he kissed my naked breasts and we laid down on the floor in each other's arms. I wanted him very much. I was curious. I kept thinking about our wedding and I told him I wanted to wait until our wedding night. He kissed me and then he got on top of me. I hugged him and we had intercourse for the first time. I found it was very enjoyable and not at all painful like they say. I had orgasms many times before we were married. But now that we are married, I don't enjoy it so much any more.

Doctor: Why is that? What is your opinion?

June: Forbidden fruit? Am I trying to punish myself subconsciously? I don't know for sure.

Doctor: Why not pretend you're *not* married? Do you think you can pretend that?

June: Oh yes. Perhaps that's the trouble with me. I've always had an excellent imagination. I was always very good at playing make believe. Perhaps that's why I still hold to these girlish ideals.

Needless to say the above discourse helped June to find her way herself. She realized that she had spent her life clinging to an ideal – that her Prince Charming would arrive and carry her – his virgin bride – away. She had experienced some guilt about surrendering to Earl and she had felt remorseful about it. She could not confront her parents without a feeling of shame. It was this feeling which brought about her frigidity. When she recognized it for what it was, she managed to laugh away her guilts and once again enjoyed sex relations with her husband.

June's postmarital frigidity might eventually have been overcome, but at the expense of her marriage, for it is doubtful that Earl, or any other man, would have tolerated such a change of response for long. On the other hand, if Earl had been more understanding, he might have recognized for himself that his task, as seducer, would be far easier if he would have romantically reminded her of their delightful love interludes shared before the marriage. Such tactful reminiscence might have overcome June's postmarital frigidity. Seduction is a two way street. It is sometimes necessary to remind a loved one that pleasure shared before can again be shared now – that words which conjure up romantic images are vital to the art of seduction.

To love is to share and trust without remorse or guilt. The key to the seduction of a bride, a fiancée, a mistress or a wife of twenty years is not easy to find. But when inhibitions are swept away, guilt and shame are likewise dispersed. All that matters is that the seducers become the seduced and the seduced become the seducers. It matters not which is which – only that love emerges triumphant in the unselfish giving of oneself to a trusted loved one. Such giving is also receiving. *Love is not found* – it is *created by lovers*.

WHEN IT COMES to a showdown the male of the species *homo sapiens* often lacks the courage to take the female in sexual surrender though she may often be willing and eager. Many young men boast continually of their sexual powers and they speak freely and at length of their numerous conquests. By Jet Set standards it is a sign of virility to be a swaggering Don Juan who has conquered dozens of beautiful girls each year. But only a few men are honest enough to admit the truth: they do not seduce as many females as they would like others to believe; and, frequently, they sometimes *never* make the bedroom scene at all. A few admit that they are not experienced and they fear the baptism of the bedroom with a young lady who has been 'swinging' with other fellows regularly. This fear is masked by a façade of courage and bravado which is, in reality, a cover up to hide deep-rooted feelings of insecurity and inadequacy. The male ego is such, particularly in the young and inexperienced, that it cannot withstand an attack on the libido. In other words, rejection of, or the spurning of an amorous advance, or a mockery of the masculinity or virility of the male can cause impotence in its many forms.

A prostitute who ridicules the size of a young man's penis may cripple his libido for life. Such a man, if he is obsessed with doubt and feelings of inadequacy, will frequently react psychologically either by becoming impotent, or by developing any number of diverse idiosyncrasies.

56

The bride who seeks to seduce her groom will do well to understand the many peculiarities of the male. She should fully understand that a man who fears impotency or who is afraid that his sex organ is inadequate may be more afraid of being ridiculed than by the necessity 'to prove' his sexual ability in bed. The wise young female who realizes this will often effect a cure that medical science cannot bring about. She will do well to remember that the male thinks of himself as a great lover whether or not he actually is. If he is not, then her words and actions can quite possibly be effective in making him into the great lover he wants to be. By removing the threat to his ego, the young lady succeeds in making him love her as he may not be capable of loving any other woman.

The following case history illustrates how it is quite possible for a young and inexperienced bride to seduce an impotent husband and help him overcome strong feelings of inadequacy.

Case No. 814
Paula S. Age 20
Subject arrived at the psychiatrist's office in obvious distress. She had been married for three months and was upset because her bridgeroom was impotent and had blamed her for his inadequacy. At first he suffered from premature ejaculation; then later, total impotency. She felt that she was 'not sexy enough' to excite him and was therefore to blame for his failure to obtain an erection. After several visits, during which times the young bride was counseled and advised in detail about what to do, she had resolved her problem. When asked what she had done, she made this statement:

'I was quite upset about my own failure to properly seduce Nate, so I guess I didn't catch on to what was expected of me at first. I'm glad you spelled it all out for me, Doctor, I hadn't known what to do and I suppose I might never have learned if I hadn't come to you for advice.

'As you know, Nate and I had only petted and necked before we were married and we had never gone all the way, so neither of us knew how it was going to be. I knew he had had lots of girls sexually and I knew he was experienced so I trusted him. He found me a virgin when we first had intercourse and he was pleased, though he was so excited that he ejaculated before he penetrated me fully. I didn't think about that because I didn't know how it was supposed to be. Later when I heard other girls talking about their first nights, I realized that perhaps Nate had reached an orgasm so fast because he was so excited and with the waiting and all, he could hardly be blamed. But later, on our honeymoon, he kept ejaculating before we could consummate our relationship. He seemed quite upset about it. He blamed me. He said he had done it to other girls for hours and hours. But he couldn't understand why he came so fast with me.

'When we came home after the honeymoon we tried to have relations but he couldn't get an erection. He was very upset and I tried to do all I could to help him, but nothing worked. I kissed him and played with his organ but that didn't help. He said that maybe I didn't excite him sexually like the other girls he had had. He swore he had never had this trouble before.

'Well, I did like you told me, Doctor. I felt his muscles and pampered his ego as best I could. I admired his physique and in particular, made a big fuss about the size of his penis. I told him that I was sure he loved me and he didn't want to hurt me with that great big thing of his. When I told him that for the first time he got very excited and we had intercourse. I told him how wonderful it was and I kept telling him how sexy he made me feel.

'I kept this up and pretty soon he was able to get an erection everytime we got into bed together. He soon overcame his problem of premature ejaculation, too. I find that now when he is down in the dumps I can bolster his ego just by kissing him and playfully fondling his organ or telling him how strong and manly he is. Sometimes I tell him how afraid I am that he'll hurt me with that big thing of his and he gets very passionate when I tell him that.

'I have found that whenever he wants sex, he now fondles and pets me too and when I respond and tell him how he excites me, he's like a tiger. We don't talk about our problems anymore because there aren't any. I love him and he loves me and I'm sure that we'll never ever leave each other on account of sex.'

This rather succinct statement clearly shows how just a little encouragement and flattery will work miracles. A woman who had been on the verge of losing her husband to whom she had been married for three years had this to say to a marriage counselor-psychologist after she had won her husband back. We quote this because this amplifies Paula's experience in the seduction art.

'I'll never be afraid of losing Victor again to another woman, Doctor, thanks to you and thanks to what I've learned from you. Actually, it was my own fault. I guess I was pretty dumb about those things. Whenever Vic wanted sex, I gave in without a fuss and tried hard to please him. I know now that all I had done was satisfy his lust, not his ego. I used to lay there and pretend I was enjoying intercourse, but I really wasn't. By the time he was finished I was just getting excited. But then it was too late. This grated on my nerves and I didn't know what to do about it.

'Then when I found out that he was having an affair with another woman, I didn't know what to do. My minister told me to see you and that's the best advice I've ever had in my life. My minister was wise enough to know that a man just doesn't cheat on his wife because he is oversexed or anything like that. It's because he isn't 'understood' at home. So when you told me that my husband was cheating on me because he found 'understanding' and appreciation in another woman's arms, I hit the ceiling at first, Doctor. Later, when I realized that what you told me was right, I examined my own ego and found out that I had a lot to learn.

'I swallowed my pride and dolled myself up like you suggested. Then I set my cap for my husband. I was determined to win him back. I was determined to forget that he had cheated on me. That wasn't easy to do. I fixed it so we could get away one weekend together when the baby was at my mother's. We went to this little town where there is a skiing lodge and we stayed there. When we went to bed I complimented him on how manly he was in his ski togs. I told him that he amazed me at how agile and muscular he was and how good he was on skis. He lapped it up.

'We were in bed talking, when I put my arm around him and touched his penis. I stroked it for the first time in my life. At least, of my own volition. I had never touched him there voluntarily before. He looked at me strangely and there was excitement in his eyes. Then I said that I thought his penis looked larger than it ever had before. He grinned and kissed me. I dug my nails into his muscles and remarked at how powerful he was and I told him that in the firelight of that skiing lodge he looked like a frontiersman. He made love to me as he had never done before. I'll tell you, Doctor, that was the most marvelous night of my life. He was vigorous and gentle, loving and brutal, all at the same time.

'I told him I couldn't get enough of his loving and I kept begging him to continue having intercourse. He had several orgasms, and so did I, for the first time in our married life. For the first time since we'd been married I had more than one orgasm in the same night. I discovered that doing the things you suggested also got me very passionate.

'The next morning, while we were under the covers, he kissed my breasts and cried like a little boy. Until that moment I had not let on that I knew he had been cheating on me. He confessed the affair. He told me that he loved me and he wanted me to forgive him; that he would never again be unfaithful. I pretended he was just an adventuresome virile guy who needed a lot of women and he wasn't to blame. That sparked his ego like something I never saw before He was a new man overnight. He loved me and it was magnificent. He'll never go away from my bed again feeling interested in another woman – thanks to what I've learned about how to seduce my man.'

Usually, a man is able to perform like a sexual gymnast with a promiscuous woman he knows he will never see again because he does not fear her soirée with him will be found out. He can feel supersexed because he is enjoying a fleeting interlude which is novel in nature. He may find that the surreptitiousness of the affair is charged with excitement and daring that titilates his ego, or he may find that he is proving himself to be a virile man by conquering a stray female. But no matter what the reason for his unfaithfulness to his wife, the chances are he is being unfaithful *because* he doesn't find adequate 'understanding' in his wife's arms. When his wife takes the time and trouble to cater to his ego, to make him feel that he is the most important guy on earth, the greatest lover, the most virile of all men, the chances are he will *not* be unfaithful to her. Of course there are extenuating circumstances. A man on a business trip, or away from his wife for a length of time, *if* he is normal and healthy, will usually *not* turn down an opportunity to go to bed with another woman. But if his wife *does* delight his ego and cater to his maleness, the odds are he will not go out of his way to find other women, even during a long absence.

The feeling of inadequacy is usually unconscious and indefinable. Many men who make a fetish of running around with other women do so because they are seeking something they themselves do not fully understand. Comprehension of *why* they need the arms of other women is important. A fully satisfied male will not seek sexual relief in the arms of strange women if he is *not* disturbed by feelings of inadequacy. When a man feels inadequate, or has some doubts about his masculinity, he will go from woman to woman seeking, not sexual satiety, but confirmation of his virility.

The foolish woman who tells her lover that his penis is not quite as 'large' as others she has had destroys his ego. A thrice-divorced woman, after entering marriage for the fourth time, made this statement to the marriage counselor who had consulted with her:

'Thank you, Doctor,' she said happily, presenting him with a cake she had baked. 'I want you to know that my fourth marriage would have been a disaster like the first three if I had not taken your wise advice. I lost those last two husbands to other women because I was stupid. I thought I was being sexy and way-out with them when I told them about my other affairs. I wanted them to think I was sexy and sought-after, but all I accomplished was driving them to the divorce courts.

'The mistake I made with my first husband, I know now, was entirely my own. I did everything but place the blame where it belonged – on myself. I thought that he wanted a mother, which explained away why he left me for an older woman. Now I know better. That older woman was a lot smarter than I was. She told him how great a lover he was and *that* did it. I never told him that. So he left me.

'The second and third marriages didn't last either because I didn't make those husbands feel adequate. I used them sexually, it is true, but I failed to reciprocate by telling them how wonderful they were.

'Now, with this man, it looks like we're going to stay married. He asked me several times if he satisfied me and you know what I told him? I told him that he was the greatest lover on earth and his penis was the biggest I had ever had, even though this wasn't quite true. He loved that and he has shown me in a thousand ways that he loves me and wants to stay married to me.

'I do other things to him which I haven't done to other men, too. I pretend I'm so excited by his manhood that I go crazy at the sight of it. He lays back upon the bed like a king and I kneel between his legs like a slave girl. I take his wand in my mouth and I kiss it like a woman worshiping at an altar.

'Just a few little tricks like this and he eats out of my hand. I never knew a man and a woman could be so sublimely happy. I would never have known this, Doctor, if I hadn't sought your advice. You've changed my life and I'll never forget it. I'm granting you permission to transcribe this statement of mine [if you promise not to reveal my real name] so that others can also benefit from the things I've learned.'

Since the times of ancient man, woman has worshiped at the altar of Priapus – the Penis God. The obelisk and the other statuary depicting the phallic symbol has stood erect since time immemorial to remind woman that if she is to hold her man, she must cater to his whims – she must worship at the altar of his manhood. If she truly shows how much she extols the virtues of his virility; if she truly shows how much she admires and appreciates his manhood; then she will succeed in seducing him and keeping him seduced.

One often wonders what some men 'see' in other women – particularly unsightly or unshapely females. The clue is in *how* that female treats her man. When asked by a psychiatrist how she had kept her actor husband for twenty-five years, a particularly homely [and overweight] matron made this statement:

'My husband is a vain guy, always has been. He's a successful actor and screen lover because he is classically handsome. Ever since he's been in show biz, which is longer than I've known him, beautiful women were after him. He may have been unfaithful occasionally, but he always came back to me. He came back to me for the same reason that I managed to steal him away from a famous actress. This, I might add, was the talk of Hollywood in those days. Nobody could figure out what he saw in me.

'That was just the point. It wasn't what he saw in me – it was the other way round. It was what *I* saw in *him*. The beauty queens and the famous starlets were competing for the spotlight of public acclaim against him. They wanted affection and adulation and were incapable of giving it. Me, I loved that guy ever since I was his script girl back at the movie lot. One day in the dressing room while I was coaching him on his lines I told him how excited he made me just to be with him. There must've been something in the way I told him that struck a chord. He looked at me and smiled and stretched across his cot and let me caress him. I felt his muscles and told him how strong he was – which was something I doubt few other women ever thought of doing or saying. He happened to be quite proud of his physique and strutted in front of me like a rooster. I started to go out with him and before you knew it, we were married.

'Every night since then I encourage him to walk around in front of me naked. Sometimes when he has some love scenes to do the next day and I know it isn't good for him to have intercourse with me before because it's tiring and sometimes it flags his interest in the romantic co-star, I find that he flips for me when I lay in bed watching him walking around naked, practicing his lines. He wants me and I want him. I'm half crazy with passion and he loves that. Now that you know my secret, do you still wonder why I've managed to hold onto him all these years?'

This statement contains the essence of the secret of seduction. A woman, just an average housewife has successfully managed to hold her strikingly handsome husband for twenty-five years without losing him to some of the most beautiful and glamorous women in America, all because she has catered to his male ego in the earthy way he needed. She knew what to say and how to say it; what to do and how to do it; and, it was all her own idea because she loved him truly enough to sense that that was *how* to win him and hold him. And in doing so she enriched her own pleasure and satisfaction.

Frequently a prudish woman or one from an overly sheltered environment or background will find herself facing the crossroads of life – what to do about an errant husband who is seeking greener pastures – and understanding, in the arms of other women. If she is able to come down to earth and realize that she needs to dismount and stay dismounted from her high horse, she may be able to reclaim her husband before he leaves her forever. If she thinks for one moment of entrapping him with those '*for the sake of the children*' or '*what will people say*' excuses she is only fooling herself. Trapped, the man returns, *sometimes*. But deep inside him the hunger still goes unsated. Deep inside his breast he feels that something is missing and his heart aches for understanding and love. He may react by turning against his wife and even his children. He may respond by becoming a tyrant or in any of a hundred or more different ways – but the fact remains that he is married in name only.

The woman who foolishly commits her husband to the no-man's land of life without fulfillment in the joy of love, also condemns herself to a barren existence. She may turn to church or social work or to a lover for fulfillment; or she may proceed to make herself as unattractive as possible to further discourage her 'loathsome' husband.

We could go on and on discussing what can happen when a woman refuses to bend a little and understand her husband; but that will accomplish less than what the discussion of what she *ought* to do will accomplish. If she thinks about herself in relation to her husband she is bound to find many things which are going awry. Is it the little things that mean and count most in life. When she looks around herself and asks, 'How have I shown my husband how much I love him?' she must find herself wanting, provided she is entirely honest. When she is able to say, 'Okay, I've done this and I've done that for him, that's not enough – I must do *more*,' she is on the right road to seduction success. Life is fraught with all kinds of problems, like those of being shortchanged in affairs; but when one realizes that happiness is ninety percent in the giving and ten percent in the getting, it is then possible to work the trick that produces happiness: start giving ninety-*nine* percent and soon a hundred percent happiness will be returning. But those who foolishly tally each giving and taking are those who are forever denied true happiness.

The wife who gazes up at her husband's face during a moment of throbbing ecstasy accomplishes *more* than does the woman who closes her eyes and moans. The look of adulation accomplishes more than words. It is an expression of love, of reverence, of appreciation. When she whispers during the ecstatic moment, 'Darling, you're the greatest – I love you – love me tender, etc.' she is *reassuring* him that he is virile and manly and her one and only, the most important guy on earth.

The delights of seduction are many and varied. But all are related. They are related to the ego. Both the male and the female ego. When the female is able to inspire the male, he in turn inspires the female – and so it goes. Each action produces a reaction. Spark ignites spark. But when something happens to douse that spark, the engine of harmony begins to miss and soon it stops running. Love and seduction are as simple, but yet, as complex, as that.

The true seductress never stops seducing; nor does the true seducer ever stop seducing the woman of his life, for instinct tells both that giving is receiving and must be constant.

At first when a couple are together the thrill of being together is yet but a novelty, and as such, it contains their interest and holds their undivided attention. But as the routine of life sets in, so does the cancer of monotony. The couple who permit their lives to become robotized and their love appetites to become jaded by routine and sameness is asking for boredom and unhappiness and disharmony to smother their lives. Just as the physical condition of the healthy body must be carefully tended with exercise, proper diet and medical care, so must the libido be titillated with variety and satiety – and new and different seduction techniques. The simple introduction of a new lovemaking technique may do the trick to whet sexual appetite. The occasional adventure of a lovemaking session in a place different from the bedroom may instill new interest and keen desire. The fun of living and the fun of loving should be revered by both parties always. Togetherness and being happy together should count most. Even when plagued by troubles and despair, a couple in love should never allow themselves to become that despondent that they put aside their togetherness or postpone their love sessions.

There is a kind of magic to life that knows no limitations. When love is kept active and jointly participated in by man and woman, all things can be resolved.

It is written that 'Love conquers all.' No truer words were ever uttered. Indeed Love *does* conquer all, and when the lover properly *seduces* lover, life itself is created.

The secret of seduction is this: it is the desire to please another with all one's heart. When either love partner truly wishes to make the other happy, the way will be found to make that happiness possible. The way to a man's heart is *not* through his stomach – it is through the phallus – the staff of life itself. Anyone who denies this has not yet learned to live or love.

NOTHING is more tragic than the disillusionment which shatters the idyllic happiness of a newlywed couple. Unfortunately, this disillusionment sometimes occurs on the first night of the honeymoon when the bride realizes there is more to marriage than a ring on her finger and a new surname. Of course, naïveté is uncommon among newlyweds of today, but shyness and timidity is quite commonplace, so much so that it appears to be one of the major problems confronting young marrieds. The fears of the wedding night are often exaggerated all out of proportion to reality. Many brides are shattered by the course of the day's events – the excitement of the marriage – the honeymoon trip, etc. – before their grooms carry them over the threshold of a new life. Hence, they are totally unprepared for what is to follow.

If the couple has not had intercourse before their wedding day, more often than not both are possessed by untold fears which they are unable to express or understand. The bride wonders if she will please her groom. The groom wonders if he will be able to perform adequately without hurting his bride. Fears, guilts, complexes and much nonsense permeates their mental states. Frequently, the aftermath of the wedding, liquor, excitement, and nervous exhaustion, takes a tremendous toll on the wits and emotional limitations of the newlyweds. This naturally is a deterrent to satisfactory 'first night' relations.

When the bride has been disillusioned, all too often she develops fixations and sexual fears which spell the end to the honeymoon at once. The consummation of the marriage was unpleasant and distasteful. It was the act which wrecked the end of a perfect day. It will be something she will never forget or forgive. Perhaps she has been unduly afraid of the expected pain when her hymen was broken. The *hymen* is the fleshy membrane situated at the mouth of the vagina which partially seals it. It usually breaks when pressure is applied, therefore gentleness is necessary if the pressure of its rupture is not to be too painful. Many women have fragile hymen strictures which do not hurt when broken; others may have rather thick hymens which cannot be broken easily or completely until the sexual act has been performed many times.

With the breaking of the hymen, all too frequently the idyll of the honeymoon is also broken. The bride finds intercourse unpleasant and painful. She is unable to respond sexually. She fails to enjoy relations, in fact, she abhors them. She has not experienced an orgasm. She is overwrought with fear and misgiving. The symbol of her virginity, which she has learned to guard with her life since childhood, has been battered asunder. She suffers a psychological shock she cannot overcome.

Many bridegrooms are likewise disappointed on the wedding night because they feel they have failed their wives. They feel they are inadequate sexually because they have not given pleasure to their wives. The fact that the bride did not respond ardently and sexually to the groom is most shattering to the male ego. Instead of beginning the marriage on the right footing, the couple stumbles into the marital union clumsily. More often than not that 'stumble' can cripple for life. Instead of happiness and bliss, unhappiness and stress encompass them. Here are some typical problems faced by couples who abruptly discovered that their honeymoons were over:

I am sure that my husband's penis is abnormally large in

*size which is the reason why I am unable to enjoy sex with
him without feeling pain. His penis, when erect, is seven
inches long and about an inch and a half in diameter. What
else can I do but ask to have our marriage annulled?*

The belief that your husband's penis is abnormal in
size when tumescent is incorrect. While it is true that the
average man's erect penis measures on an average from
five inches to slightly over seven inches, it is also true that
occasionally intercourse is painful, regardless of the size of
the male organ when the woman's vagina is unusually
small or is blocked by the unbroken hymen. Before taking
any drastic measures to end your marriage, it is important
that both you and your husband submit to physical examinations by a medical doctor. Frequently, it has been
learned that painful intercourse is the result of improper
lubrication of the penis and vagina prior to intercourse.
Usually this occurs when there is an absence of preliminary foreplay which generally arouses the sex organs
to a state of excitability wherein the vagina and penis are
lubricated naturally by secretions from the body. Often,
in newly-wed couples, intercourse is painful to the bride
because her hymen may be ruptured only partially, hence
making intercourse unpleasant. A competent physician
will correct any difficulty such as this in a matter of minutes.
The use of jelly lubricants are also recommended.

The vagina in the average woman is so constructed that
it will stretch sufficiently to admit the average-sized penis.
Not infrequently the complaint registered by many women
is that their vaginas are too large and their husbands'
penes, too small. Very often young brides are overly
apprehensive about the size of their husbands' organs.
This concern is only natural and can be dispelled by commonsense explanation. Most libraries and bookstores today have numerous volumes to lend or sell which deal with
detailed explanations of the size, shape, and peculiarities
of male and female reproductive organs. Ignorance is not
bliss – it is frequently distressing and painful – so avail your-

self of the knowledge which abounds around you and consult a qualified marriage counselor or physician.

My husband is impotent. He cannot get an erection now that we are married, though he was always able to do so when we petted and occasionally had intercourse before our wedding. Is God punishing us for being indiscreet before we got married? We are both very religious and our clergymen told us that that was why he was impotent.

The chances are that your husband is impotent because of the guilt feelings he has no doubt acquired as a result of his religious training. No, 'God' does not punish people for being intimate with each other. When someone tries to tell you this, you can rest assured that person is ignorant and unqualified to so inform you, for nothing is more false. Impotency is usually a state of mind. Usually it is due to a psychological conflict which can be resolved with competent psychological help.

According to Kinsey, more than fifty percent of all men and women had premarital intercourse before they were married. Such being the rule rather than the exception, you are not alone.

Actually, the fact that you and your husband obviously indulged in sexual intercourse before your marriage on a 'catch as catch can' basis had much to do with his potency – and your pleasure – *then* because of the very surreptitious nature of your lovemaking. A quality of excitement and novelty was present before you were married which is now absent after you have married. The psychological stimulation you both shared prior to married life was, of course, of an erotic nature. Now that is missing. Now you can legally go to bed together. Consequently, your husband is impotent because the aura of excitement is now gone and that has been replaced with his preconscious guilt feelings. Do talk your problem over carefully. All that matters is that you both love each other and wish to make each other happy. Do not scoff at him or deride him in any way because of his temporary deficiency. In time he will overcome it, provided of course, he understands the reason why he is impotent.

Occasionally couples are able to recapture some of their premarital sexual interludes by having coitus away from home in some trysting place similar to those visited before marriage.

Very rarely, however, impotency in males results from physical ailments. It is always wise to consult a physician, but quite unwise to consult someone who is unqualified to give adequate advice.

My husband is a worrier. He is always overly concerned about the pleasure he is giving me during the sex act. He reaches orgasm quickly, long before I am ready. How can I tell him, without hurting him, that he is not satisfying me? I realize that if I tell him this, he may become totally impotent.

You are wise in considering what effect the truth might have upon your husband. However, there are remedies which may be taken that will work miracles. They are the remedies that only you, as a wife, can give him. The first thing to do is try to understand why your husband is trying so hard to please you. When you think about this you will discover that he is really quite afraid and rather unsure of himself. He seeks assurance from you because he is overly concerned about his own virility and needs constant *reassurance*. Only you can give him this reassurance. You must flatter him and bolster his ego. It is wise to tell him that he is exciting and masculine and that his organ is so large it both frightens and excites you. The woman who tells her husband that she loves him and then begs him to be gentle with her and to make love to her with his huge sex organ is a woman who seduces her husband into being the man that he would be – rather

72

than the man that he is *afraid* he cannot be.

The fact that your husband is a 'worrier' is indicative that he is quite insecure and unsure of his manliness. You would do well to help him overcome this psychological weakness.

He loves you and wants to satisfy you, but is afraid he will fail. It is the fear of failure alone that renders most men impotent. The fear of ridicule because of sexual failure is the second major cause of male impotence. Assure your husband the honeymoon is *not* over. Try your best to overcome his fears and do give him the self-confidence he needs.

The female counterpart of the male 'worrier' is frequently seen as the woman who continually frets over her sexual performance and must ask over and over whether or not she is pleasing her husband. She needs reassurance because she is basically insecure. She must be told she is beautiful and sexy. She cannot go for long without reassurance that she is lovely and loved. The problems faced by these people are deep-rooted, having originated early in childhood. Hence, one cannot expect that such problems can be swiftly overcome in a few hours or weeks, or even months, for that matter, because what has taken years and years to form must be painstakingly *un*formed by diligent, professional or skilled help.

Now that I'm married, I am convinced that I made a mistake. My wife is beautiful and talented, but I thought I was marrying a 'good' girl and a virgin – instead it turned out that she wasn't a virgin. What should I do, divorce her?

You are typical of many young men with erroneous ideas about what constitutes a 'good' girl and what constitutes a 'bad' one. In the first place, you are starting your marriage off on the wrong foot because you still cling to false 'ideals' concerning the realities of life. Actually, you are angry because your bride did not surrender to you sexually before you were married. [This was determined after further questioning of the subject.] You used as a basis to 'test' the goodness or badness of the girls you dated a deception – you figured that any girl that you could seduce was therefore 'bad' and not eligible to marry you. On the other hand, you reasoned that any girl you could not seduce, you knew to be 'good'.

By rights, you have been busy deceiving girls all during your youth, therefore you have set yourself up as a self-styled 'expert' and moralist. You have decided that you alone are righteous and all the world is wrong. Wake up and stop being a hypocrite, will you? If you loved the girl well enough to wish to marry her, and if you did, does the fact that she lost her virginity when she was a teenager really make her 'bad' for that juvenile mistake? Love her and forgive her. You aren't alone.

When you went on your search to find a bride for yourself did you ask every girl you dated, 'Let's go to bed. I want to test you to see if you're a virgin. If you're not, then I don't wish to consider you for marriage'. Or did you falsely allude to being 'in love' with the girls you dated and then deceive them into surrendering to you because you led them to believe you were going to marry them? In either case, you were only kidding yourself. This girl or that one is or isn't 'nice' according to your yardstick.

You are typical of many immature men, individuals who have reached physical maturity, but have failed to grow up emotionally and intellectually. Because of people like you in both sexes, much unhappiness is caused and many good people are injured permanently.

When people such as you marry, you fail to recognize that those who fall in love with you and marry you, *trust* you. Girls by nature wish to be loved and petted. Such individuals are easily duped. A trusting young lady will usually surrender herself if she believes it is necessary to do so in order to hold the man she has grown to love. The man who dupes such a girl and slakes his lust on her with no thought for her whatsoever is a heel and a cad in this book.

But most men, when they go after sexual conquests, create an emotional wall between themselves and their sex partners. They seek only to get as close as possible physically, but they refuse to allow themselves to 'fall in love' or become emotionally entangled. When men have lived by this practice it usually is quite difficult for them to remove the wall when they do meet a woman they wish to marry. To their shock and surprise, these individuals learn too late that they have built a wall around themselves which forever forbids them from becoming emotionally 'involved' with any woman. Then they express their dismay that 'I just can't find a decent girl to marry', and they rationalize that there is safety in one sexual relationship after another and they therefore doom themselves to lives of promiscuity and emptiness. The roué and the Don Juan may have all the answers about the techniques of the sex act, but if he has been habitually deceitful and selfish in his sexual adventures, he may have acquired a mountain of troubles and worries about finding a woman he can really love. He never learns that love is not found, but made . . . he misconstrues the 'how' of making love as a mechanical device of pleasure.

Since I've been married I've been worried that my husband and I have been having sex relations too much. Sometimes we make love two and three times a day. We've been married one year now and I'm afraid that we're going to become sex fiends or something. Am I correct in this assumption?

The real difficulty lies in the attitude your husband and you have concerning sex. If you are equally desirous of frequent relations and are physically able to enjoy same, more power to you, for there is nothing harmful or wrong in having coitus on an average of once or twice a day. However, if you are developing feelings of sex guilt, you

75

may be doing yourself drastic harm, for nothing is more destructive physically or emotionally than anxiety and guilt which is allowed to build up within oneself. Of course, not everyone who suffers from a sense of guilt suffers irreparable harm to the psyche. Many people gradually overcome their feelings of guilt in time and by commonsense. Most people who are stricken with feelings of guilt eventually overcome them; a few do not. When this happens it is wise to search for the causes. Sometimes it is good to consider that everybody else does the same thing, although perhaps not as frequently. Then again, there are others who indulge in sex activities more frequently than you have mentioned.

Frequently, individuals worry too much about the methods of sexual contact they practice. Many fictitious stories evolve around the consequences of oral-genital relations and other forms of lovemaking. It is wise not to believe what you hear – just do what comes naturally and what you enjoy.

The types of sex behavior and frequency of relations vary from society to society. In some parts of the world, coitus is engaged in plurally with no thought of the consequences. In other parts of the world the sanctity of intimate relations is held sacred. Practically all people everywhere at one time or another indulge in activity which their peers consider to be unwholesome. Whatever you do, don't worry about what others say. The chances are they do not know what they are talking about.

I'm afraid that my husband doesn't truly love me. I think he married me only because he was sexually attracted to me. How can I tell if he really loves me instead of the sex I give to him? Can I 'test' him by denying him my favors?

There is no test that determines how much a man loves a woman from which sex relations may be subtracted or added as plus or minus factors. If you are seeking to 'prove'

76

to yourself that your husband loves you for yourself alone – without sex – you are making the fatal mistake that so many other immature, insecure young women commit. You are saying without being blunt that you consider sexual relations as a thing apart from marital relations and man-woman love. This is the immature individual's way of looking at love and sex. You cannot 'test' your husband by denying him your favors, for in so doing you will be denying him your love. The truth is, love and sex *are* inseparable in a mature adult relationship.

If your husband approaches you crudely, without making love to you and without the usual preliminaries, of course you are entitled to wonder if he truly loves you or merely lusts after you. But – if you are a mature adult, and if you are capable of communicating with your husband, then you must do what so many millions of other women do in your situation – you *must* be loving and understanding and receptive to him. When you take the initiative and when *you* seduce him, he will naturally reciprocate. But if you protest and try to evade him, instead of being loving and understanding, you are being just the opposite. You are rejecting him. When a man – or woman, for that matter, is constantly rejected, and when complaints instead of compliments are heard, is there any wonder that sex relations become a physical encounter sans the romantic aspects of it?

There is only one way to be sure of your husband's love – make love to him, be seductive in every way you can. When he responds, in all ways, then you will know.

At times our sex relations are dull and unexciting. How can my husband and I increase our sex satisfaction?

Erotic stimulation is the key to satisfactory and enjoyable sex relations. When practiced with a view to seducing the sex partner, and when that mutuality is shared, sex relations *are* naturally more enjoyable and satisfactory.

77

However, there are times when other steps must be taken in order to increase sexual gratification and to heighten sensation.

One of these times occurs frequently after childbirth, when the vaginal muscles are lax as the result of child-bearing. Many women suffer from this problem. They are unable to control the vaginal muscle. When control is lacking, of course the woman will experience little satisfaction from coitus. Often she will become frigid.

This form of genital relaxation often occurs at all ages. The muscle is a double band which surrounds the openings of the vagina, urethra and anus in the pelvic floor. It stretches from the tip end of the spine to the front bone of the pelvis. When it becomes flabby and weak or is thinly developed, it fails to hold the pelvic organs in place. Several world-famous gynecologists have developed methods for strengthening this muscle. If such is the problem in your instance, it will be wise to consult your physician. Once the muscle tone has been restored, the vaginal muscles can once again respond to coitus enjoyably and give pleasure to both partners.

Often, a variation of the sex act is sufficient to heighten sexual pleasure. Be sure you have tried them all.

I am afraid that I am frigid. I cannot attain an orgasm every time my husband and I have intercourse. What can I do?

Contrary to popular misconception, the female orgasm is quite different from the male orgasm. There is no noticeable discharge of fluid such as when the man ejaculates. Moreover, the construction of the female genitals in which the clitoris is partly concealed makes it difficult at times for contact or friction between the penis and the clitoris to take place. For this reason, the female is often denied the full measure of satisfaction which the male enjoys. It is largely up to the male to make certain he is

78

adequately gratifying the female.

Moreover, too much emphasis is placed on the need for an orgasm each time intercourse is had. While it is true that the man must expend his semen in order to obtain relief, it is likewise true that the woman need not reach an orgasm to obtain satisfaction from the love act. In the past, most married men were accused of being concerned only with their own orgasm. Gradually, as sexual equality freed the woman from the old sex taboos, the husbands learned to take their wives' needs into consideration too. Today it is a matter of common knowledge that both man and woman are entitled to equal sexual rights – and man is *expected* to see to it that his wife is gratified.

Many husbands, when unable to bring their wives to orgasm through normal intercourse, frequently resort to manipulation of the female organ with finger or tongue, or new variations in sexual positions are tried. The lover who makes certain that he is pleasing his partner is one who is always sure to be gratified in return. The fear of being 'frigid' is often worse than frigidity itself. When understanding and patience is exercised, no such thing as frigidity exists.

The honeymoon need never be over when a couple take the time and the trouble to seduce each other – and then continue to show consideration and love for each other. As it has been pointed out previously several times, seduction is frequently a state of mind – whether it is a nightmare or a blissful dream, is up to the individual.

Seduction As A Way of Life

WHEN A HOUSEWIFE runs to answer the doorbell she pauses before opening the door to put on lipstick and pat her hair in place. Who knows, but some handsome salesman might be calling and she wants to look 'nice'.

When an old married man gallantly stops his car to give aid to a lady motorist with a flat tyre, before getting out he usually glances at his reflection in the rearview mirror to make certain he looks well groomed and, perhaps, 'attractive'.

In fact, everyone wants to look 'attractive'.

Why?

Why all the stress on being 'attractive'? Does this mean the same as being well groomed, handsome, beautiful, nice to look at? No. It means exactly what the word means – attractive to the opposite sex. This need for being 'attractive' is inbred into the human personality. In fact, everything in society from early childhood to death is oriented toward 'attractiveness'. All emphasis is placed upon looking one's best at all times. The youngest children are extremely conscious or the clothing they wear and the styles of dress. Newspaper advertisements, magazine ads, radio and television commercials, all heavily emphasize the 'attractiveness' of the goods being offered for sale, *and* the attractiveness of the attractive people who benefit from or use those goods and services. Commercials extolling the virtues of deodorants, cigarettes, beer, soap and automobiles place heavy emphasis on the 'attractiveness' of people who use those products. Even some automobile commercials are so bold as to suggest that individuals who drive the latest model Blooper Eight are 'sexy' and 'attractive'.

The stereotyped society we live in today places all emphasis on an image of 'attractiveness'. What was obscene and unmentionable five decades ago is now 'in'. At one time it was disgraceful to display a feminine undergarment in public – today it is quite the thing. At one time the woman who smoked in public was looked upon with disdain – today she is 'in'. In fact, she is not 'in' if she does not conform by using the latest fadist cosmetic or 225 calorie luncheon drink.

The age of the bikini is upon us. Women are no longer frowned upon for displaying their legs or painting their lips.

Why?

Seduction has become *the* way of life. You are not 'in' if you fail to be attractive to others. In other words, if you are not sexually attractive, you don't count. Marriage is no longer the institution it once was. Today's modern housewife dresses to look her best – her seductive best. Men with roving eyes may look all they want, but they're not supposed to touch. Ridiculous? Of course. Why go to all that trouble to look enticing, alluring, glamorous, and seductive if you have no intention of permitting liberties to the men you attract? Some apologists maintain that women dress for other women. How silly can you get? Unless you mean that these women who dress to outdo other women are not trying to attract them, but rather, to make them envious. Why?

So what if another person is jealous of what you possess, or flaunt, or the way you look. Does this add to your life? Except for inflation of the ego, such vanity has no purpose whatsoever.

The man who takes care of himself physically by exercise, diet, etc. usually does so because he wants others to admire him; so it is with the female counterpart. But why bother to seduce others if there is no intent to follow through? This is puzzling to some, but hilarious to others. And then there are some who need a boost to the ego in order to feel desirable and wanted. Such is the way of modern life.

That housewife who primps before she opens the door to receive a male caller will deny emphatically that she powdered her nose and put on fresh lipstick before admitting the salesman just because it was her intention to seduce him. She will aver that her only intent was to look 'presentable'. Yet, she appears before the caller, her face carefully made up, her hair neatly groomed. Why? For what purpose? Why did she go to all that trouble just to receive a stranger she has never before met? Is she unhappily married? Is she planning to take a lover and be unfaithful to her husband? Does she need admiration and love and attention? Does she hope to obtain all these things from a mere stranger? Perhaps she does. Perhaps down deep within her unconscious she hopes that the stranger calling at her door will sweep her off her feet and carry her off on a white stallion. She will deny this, of course, but secretly she knows – though she is usually unable to admit it even to herself – that she secretly *does* wish to seduce the stranger. The proof is in the doing. She primps and tries to look attractive for the stranger, *but* she does not apply fresh makeup or change into something flattering to be attractive for her husband when *he* comes home. Why?

A good question.

She has the husband all the time. She is used to him. She is certain of him. She has a piece of paper – a marriage license. Therefore, she doesn't have to seduce him. She only must seduce strangers – but *not* for the purpose of enticing them to go to bed with her.

The roué who helps the stranded motorist fancies himself as quite a charmer and he is quick to make overtures to the lady in distress. According to Kinsey, better than thirty percent of all married men engage in extramarital relations. Better than twenty-five percent of all married women engage in extramarital sex relations. Therefore is it any wonder that so much emphasis is placed upon the need for looking attractive to members of the opposite sex?

The human psyche is such that few people really ever fully understand themselves. It is difficult to resolve egoistic needs and conform them to the proprietary restrictions of society. Man is indeed a polygamous animal, but is this because his ego is such that he needs to 'prove' his masculinity again and again? Is he tempted by 'attractive' women in miniskirts who display themselves to him provocatively, or would he *not* be tempted if the entire female society around him ceased their efforts to attract him and every other man in the street? Does modern man cheat on his wife and be unfaithful to his mistress because it is 'the thing to do', or is he tempted because the sight of so many seductively attired females everywhere he goes has kept him in a perpetually excited state?

Man is voyeuristic. He enjoys looking, especially at attractive women. But he will also look if they are not pretty by usual standards. He watches breasts, buttocks, faces, legs. He is fascinated by the size of breasts and buttocks. He stares at knees. He will crane his neck to watch a woman undress if perchance her window blind is up. All his life, from childhood on, man is a peeper. He goes to great lengths to see what is enticingly concealed from him. He is intrigued by the packaging and the alluring makeup and the seductive perfumery; hence, he is continually tempted to *look*.

The courts throughout America are plagued with the problem of what to do with the countless thousands of Peeping Toms who are arrested each year for looking in windows and through keyholes. The Peeping Tom is everywhere, inspired by the exhibitionistic attire and behavior of girls and women. But hardly a girl or woman is arrested for 'peeping' or 'indecent behavior' except of course when they are taken into custody at burlesque shows. The 'image makers' on Madison Avenue do their best to encourage sexiness and attractiveness with little regard to the consequences of such tawdriness. Instead of emphasizing the merits of a product they are touting, it is more acceptable to emphasize sex because, as everyone knows, *sex sells*.

With the advent of the 'mod' styles, women did not protest when it became quite the rage to wear skin tight pants or miniskirts even though these same women, a few years before, would not have allowed themselves to be seen in public with so much of their anatomy revealed for all to see. Seduction is a 'happening' that takes place everywhere, in the food market, the theater, the club, on the street. Girls and housewives on the way to the shopping center, with their hair done up in curlers, parade around saucily attired in bikini shorts with open midriffs and peekaboo blouses; then they wonder why men make passes – even at those who wear glasses. Why else would a woman so seductively display herself, if not to attract the male? This paradox of human behavior is difficult for the male to understand. He may be a salesman or a gas station attendant. He may be a good husband and father; yet, when he sees a half naked female, no matter how homely she is, that old sex urge is awakened within him.

Psychologists and psychiatrists have written and publicly stated time and again that all too frequently man is unable to concentrate on his career or his chores because he is beset with a craving for sexual gratification. He is plagued by the sight of attractive females whose charms are enticingly concealed who surround him on the job, in the office, in the restaurant, and on the street. In fact, 'girl watching' has become quite the thing for men of all ages. Hardly a man anywhere will not stop what he is doing to watch an attractive girl sashay by, waggling her buttocks and jiggling her breasts. Because he is kept in such a permanent state of sexual awareness, naturally his consciousness is fogged with constant thoughts of sexuality. Eroticism is everywhere today. The cosmeticians and the clothiers and the beauty consultants have succeeded in overselling the public on the attributes of looking attractive. With so much attention on vanity, is there any wonder why so little heed has been paid to things which are more important and vital to humanity?

Seduction no longer concerns itself solely with enticing the affectionate love of a dear one – it has become a way of life that lures men and women away from their homes and families. The emotionally immature and the psychologically insecure are the first ones to be enticed away from their mates. Relatively many people today engage in frivolous flirtations – the majority of people enjoy tempting and seducing the 'Joneses' without giving thought to the consequences. Conversely, too few married couples today emphasize the importance of focusing their seductive efforts on their mates. The grass in the neighbor's backyard looks much greener than their own. More marriages are broken up today because the partners are victimized by the image of mass sexuality which is foisted on the public. Large numbers of men and women acquire false ideals of what love and seduction and life are all about. Desire is whetted by the unrelenting focus on sexuality and when opportunity presents itself, an affair is entered into. Love is the excuse, but curiosity the reason.

In a large eastern city recently, a married man made a date with a fifty dollar call girl who lives in a posh apartment building. He could only sneak out to see her in the morning before going to work. The girl, whose profession kept her out all night, consented to meet him one morning. 'I'll leave my door unlocked, honey,' she said. 'Just come up, get undressed, and get into bed with me. I'll know you're there and we'll have a go at it, okay?'

He agreed. The morning arrived for his date. He could not kiss his wife goodbye because he was guilt-ridden. In order to bolster his courage to keep the rendezvous, which was to be the first extramarital affair he was to have in fifteen years of marriage, he had been argumentive with his wife. He had deliberately picked a quarrel with her over some nonsensical thing in order to justify to himself what he was planning to do.

He parked his car around the corner from the girl's apartment building. Then he entered an elevator and rode up two floors above her apartment so no one would know that he was going to see that particular call girl, although he was unknown in the building, and more than three hundred tenants resided there. He got off two floors above the girl's apartment, then walked down the fire exit. He crept along the carpeted hallway until he reached the girl's door. He opened the door and went inside. In a sumptuous bed, fast asleep, was the girl he had never seen before. She was enticingly dressed in a black lace baby doll pajama outfit. Her blonde hair was attractively arranged on the pillow. He entered the bedroom, undressed, and got into bed beside her. Then, just as he was about to put his arm around her and kiss her, the thought suddenly occurred to him: 'Suppose I'm in the wrong apartment? Suppose this isn't the girl I made the date with on the phone? Suppose the door is open because the girl is expecting her husband or boy friend? Suppose that husband or boy friend comes in with a gun?'

With that, the businessman got up, dressed hurriedly, and left.

Two weeks later he went to see a psychiatrist. While his virility had never before been in question, now he had a problem. He was unable to get an erection. He had become totally impotent with his wife. He wanted to know why.

After several visits to the psychiatrist, he learned why. The psychiatrist smiled and said, 'I've heard of men being scared stiff before – but this is the first time I've heard of a case where a man was scared soft!'

The tragic humor of the experience dawned on him. He burst into laughter. He realized that he indeed had been frightened out of his wits. For the first time he realized how much his wife's respect and love for him meant and he had been obsessed with guilt – and fear – because of what *might* have happened if his imagined fantasies had been real. He had been toying with the idea of cheating on his wife for a long time. Not because his wife did not satisfy him sexually, but rather because he had been hankering to go to bed with another woman – any woman. They all looked so seductive and enticing to him that he had begun to get the idea that he was missing something. But what? He did not know; hence, he chose to try going to bed with someone else.

There is a contrast to this true story which actually happened to a young wife in a large southern city last year. Although happily married and adequately satisfied sexually, this pretty young woman felt herself attracted to the owner of a local hardware store. She wondered how it would be if she took him as a lover. Eventually, after several years of wondering, an opportunity arose wherein she found herself alone in the home with said hardware store proprietor. The man had personally delivered a few items she had purchased and she thanked him by offering him a drink. While they sat chatting over their glasses of liquor, she enticingly displayed her shapely legs. The hardware man took the liberty of touching her thighs, she put up a feeble battle and they ended up in bed. Normally, with her husband, the young woman usually always enjoyed sex relations, usually obtaining an orgasm, too. But with the casual lovemaking partner she found that she did not enjoy coitus. She froze up, in fact. Thoughts of what might happen if her husband came home early from the job; of what might happen if one of her neighbors had seen the hardware man enter the house staying longer than necessary; occured to her.

She too wound up in a psychiatrist's office a few weeks later. Her problem? She had become totally frigid and was no longer able to enjoy sexual intercourse with her husband. He insisted that she see a psychiatrist.

When the story of her affair eventually was admitted to the physician, the young woman suddenly realized that her troubles began on the day she had first been unfaithful to her husband.

87

'I guess,' she said wryly, her face coloring noticeably, 'this is just a case of curiosity killing the cat, isn't it?'

The psychiatrist smiled and nodded. He explained that her guilt had rendered her frigid. He explained how her subconscious anxiety had affected her emotions. Now that the problem was out in the open, it could be rationalized intelligently. She did so, and was no longer frigid. Though she felt the inclination to confess her affair to her husband, she decided against it because she realized it would hurt him terribly. Since then she has been a loyal wife and a better sex partner.

Casual affairs similar to the two cases just presented are more frequent today than at any other time in history because society is freer, and seduction has become a way of life. Too few people actually believe they are truly happy. They see 'attractive' people everywhere around themselves and they long to know them intimately.

The picture of a sexy model on a billboard is enough to inflame the senses of a boy or man who feels the need for sexual gratification. A commercial on television, extolling the virtues of a vacation resort, displays the saucy buttocks of a pert young girl in a bikini. There is no doubt that more than one single or married man has become unduly excited at the enticing sight of that girl's backside. A psychiatrist told this author that he had at least three male patients who admitted becoming so sexually aroused at the sight of half nude women on television that they were compelled to masturbate while seated in their armchairs at home.

Is such a way of life healthy? It is for the emotionally mature and the psychologically healthy; but it is conducive to an *un*healthy frame of mental health in those who are immature. The individual with the personality disorder will frequently be inspired to do socially unacceptable things in order to gratify his inflamed desire. The exhibitionist, upon seeing a naked thigh of a woman seated on a bus may be compelled to exhibit himself to her, for such a sight excites him and he only knows one way to relieve himself. The Peeping Tom, the child molester, and other sexually unstable individuals are prompted to react when they too are incensed by what they see everywhere around them. For example, there is a suntan lotion advertisement which depicts a little girl whose panties are being pulled down by a puppy. Her rounded buttocks are exposed. A child molester, arrested in a large southern city in 1967, admitted to the court psychiatrist that he had been unable to control his impulse to molest a seven year old little girl after seeing this advertisement on television. In fact, he admitted that the ad excited him everytime he saw it. We wonder how many other deviates there are who are similarly seduced by such advertisements which range from bra and girdle ads to soda pop commercials.

Too much attention is placed upon beauty and attracting others and too little attention is focused on the art of being faithful and endearing to one's loved ones. Consequently, the newlyweds who are blissfully happy at first, become dissatisfied with their lot and they look to others for what they 'imagine' they are being denied at home. Society inflicts upon those who live within it some crassly hypocritical demands. People falsely identify themselves with unrealistic 'ideals'. Movie stars and matinee idols set the pace for public behavior. All is sham because life is anything *but* the way it is portrayed in films and in publicity stories.

Divorces are prevalent because men and women are not taught how to live with one another, not to mention living with themselves. Instead of adjusting to one another, couples seek solace elsewhere. Men and women hunt for the unobtainable in a tinsel society. Reality has given way to pretense and falseness. Grey-haired men are blonds and brunettes, their age concealed from the women they would seduce. Brown-haired women are blondes; straight-haired women have curls, flat chested women have falsified bosoms, narrow shouldered men have padded shoulders, short men affect elevator shoes – all is an illusion. Reality has given way to unreality.

But the truth of seduction lies not in creating a false image, but in sincerity and enthusiastic avowal of affection. The true happiness is to be found only by those who practice the art of seduction with their loved ones. The seducers who are sincere not only 'attract' the seducees, but they as well continue their practice of the art of seduction to *hold* the persons they love enough to keep seduced.

Seduction in Childhood:
Unintentional Seduction

PSYCHOLOGISTS and psychiatrists the world over have agreed that the basis for adult emotional and mental illness frequently is established early in life. The tender years of childhood are those during which the individual is most vulnerable to influence. When stress or environmental pressures are exerted against the immature child, anxiety states arise. If allowed to persist, disorders of the nervous system, character disorders, and personality disturbances occur. Unfortunately the average layman cannot detect a budding disturbance of emotional origin in a child because, as is usually the case, the child is too near or dear. 'Oh he'll stop throwing those tantrums,' or, 'She's just a little high-strung and she'll soon grow out of that,' are typical remarks uttered by parents, relatives, friends, and teachers of children who misbehave or 'act up'.

But little do the well-meaning adults surrounding the disobedient or 'nervous' child realize that temper tantrums and mischievous acts really are symptoms of deeper emotional disturbances. At times the child cannot get along with his peers, or his brothers and sisters. He must fight to assert himself. He must battle for equal rights. He must compete for the love of a parent. And if he fails to play the game as well as the next child, and if he is unable to achieve the same high level of school grades as his rivals, he suffers feelings of inferiority.

Most of the time, unfortunately, the older children or adults around the child are to blame for his budding state of emotional instability. The disciplinarian who in childhood.

A child is naturally curious about sexual matters. Consequently, he often goes to great lengths to learn all he can about sex. Much of what he learns on his own initiative is erroneous. Sometimes he or she can be irreparably harmed for life by experiences encountered during the formative years of childhood. Sometimes the child is victimized by older children, or by adults. At times he may be victimized deliberately. At other times, unintentionally or unwittingly.

But when a child has been seduced by an older child or an adult, often he or she may suffer enormously as a result. The most common offense against children is that of unintentional seduction.

The parent of the opposite sex who permits her son to see her nude or who unwittingly exposes herself before the child is the most frequent offender. Either his upbringing or her attempt to be 'modern' are to blame for her careless behavior. Little does she know that even at the tender age of three years, a little boy is keenly aware of sex differences between boys and girls. Little does she realize that a little boy who takes liberties with his mother's body *does* know what he is doing – and, she is in a way contributing to his budding forwardness, if not seducing him unwittingly.

The child who witnesses the act of coitus, or who watches his parents caress each other intimately, more often than not is deeply disturbed by what he or she has seen. The mother who continues to bathe her son until almost the age of puberty very often stirs him sexually without being aware of what she is doing.

The case of a young man of eighteen years who was sentenced to prison for attempted rape shows what happens when a boy has been unwittingly seduced by his mother at a tender age. Here are the details of that case in the subject's own words as transcribed by the prison psychologist.

That night she told my father what had happened. I was listening at the door. He called me a dirty name and was going to give me a beating, but my mother stopped him.

'I'll never forget as long as I live how excited I was when I achieved that orgasm in her hand. It was the first time anybody else had ever touched me down there when I had a hard penis. I used to masturbate and think of my mother doing that to me.

'When I was sixteen she died and I ran away from home because the old man and I never did get along real well. I then started doing some handyman work and odd jobs for women around town. Some of them were real nice to me and a couple of them let me go to bed with them.

'I didn't realize it at the time, but I had this terrible urge to find a woman that was like my mother. I knew it was wrong to think of my mother that way, but I couldn't help myself. Especially when I wanted relief. I couldn't make it with girls my own age – I guess because I was afraid of them or something. I used to figure that older women were experienced and more sexy.

'One night after I had finished painting a fence for this woman I asked her if it was okay if I used her bathroom to wash up. She said, sure, so I went up stairs and got undressed. I got real excited because something reminded me of that feeling I'd had when I was a kid, that time when my mother held my penis when I was ejaculating.

'I called out to the woman and asked her if she wouldn't mind washing my back. She laughed and said why not, she had a son older than me and it might be fun. She came in and got down on her knees beside the tub. I got so excited that I couldn't wait for her to scrub me down there, so I grabbed her hand and put it on my penis. She held it for a minute and I thought I saw her get excited too, so I jumped up and pulled up her dress. She started to yell and I held her and tried to have relations with her, but she turned putting her bare backside to me. I thought that was a sign that she wanted sex too, coming up there to wash me in the tub, and then not wearing any panties,

95

so I stuck my penis in her backside and the second I felt my skin touch her, I ejaculated. She ran out of the room screaming. The neighbors heard the commotion, called the cops, and the cops caught me running out of the kitchen door.'

Of course John M.'s story has been greatly abbreviated to show the *effects* of unwitting parental seduction on a young child. The fixation John had on his mother was aggravated by an unhappy home life and conflict with a brutal father. His growing neurotic behavior and the fixation on sex culminated before the incident in the bathtub when he ejaculated in his mother's hand. But the incident itself triggered intense guilt and shame feelings that he was unable to cope with. He dropped out of school. He could not get along with children of his own age. He felt inadequate and was shy with girls. His incestuous feelings toward his mother intensified after the encounter in the tub. He punished himself by thinking of it and at the same time he derived satisfaction by recalling the event while he masturbated. His limited experience in sexual matters, the guilt about excessive masturbation, the fear of his father, the shame that his father knew what he had done – all this distorted his emotional growth. Thus he became fixated on the mother-object. He could only find satisfaction with an older woman, one who reminded him of his mother.

John M. received some limited psychotherapy from the prison psychiatrist. He was a model prisoner and was paroled after serving two years. The parole officer reported that John has settled down and married – a woman twenty years his senior. The psychiatrist feels that he will eventually mature and his wife will give him the motherly attention he needs.

The case of Bernard S. is another true example of what happens by unwitting parental seductive behavior. Here is a brief transcript of that case history:

Case No. 942
Bernard S. Age 36
Sentenced to one year for prowling and indecent behavior.

'. . . I don't know why I got this urge to peek in women's bedroom windows, except that it's the only way I can find relief. I suppose I'm oversexed. I guess I always have been oversexed, even when I was a kid. I used to see my mother in the bathroom or in the bedroom without any clothes on and she used to laugh at me and run and hide. I was around thirteen, I guess, when I watched her take a douche in the bathroom. I was hiding in the shower with the curtain pulled around me and while she was douching she peeked in the curtain and laughed, calling me a dirty-minded boy. I had this hole in my pants pocket and I was holding myself when she said that and I came in my hand. It was very exciting.

'Later, I used to peek in the keyhole and sometimes I'd hide behind the door and watch my mother through the crack. I used to masturbate a lot and I couldn't think of anything else except sex.

'Then we moved to an apartment house and I used to peek across the court at the windows of the women who lived there. Sometimes they would walk around stark naked and that drove me out of my mind. Once I masturbated eight times in one night watching this couple have intercourse.

'I don't know what got me started thinking about watching people, but I used to get my biggest thrill out of watching my mother. I never did know if she knew I was watching her, but I sort of got the idea that she knew I was and she got a charge out of it.'

Bernard S.'s troubles began when he was five. His mother divorced his father and there followed a succession of lovers. Bernard admitted this much later, although he deigned from speaking openly about it at first to the therapist. He fancied himself in the role of his mother's lover – a carryover from the normal Oedipal phase of prepuberty. He was insecure and often alone as a child. He developed slowly and did not mingle with his peers. He acquired the habit of masturbation at an early age. He feels inadequate and is latently homosexual. His voyeurism is a substitute for sexual relations; a phantasy which accompanies his compulsive masturbation. He was not responsive to therapy. Since his initial arrest at age twenty-three for prowling and voyeurism, he has been imprisoned five times. It is felt that the unintentional seduction of his mother who exhibited her nude and partially nude body to him during his formative years was the main contributing factor of his sexual aberration. He is in need of long term psychotherapy but this is not available to him because he is unwilling to make sacrifices to bear the cost.

This case of Emily R. graphically shows what happens when a girl of seven is unintentionally seduced by her father.

Case No. 354
Emily R. Age 17
Committed to state psychiatric hospital for an indefinite period. Suicidal tendencies.

Emily R. is a pretty teenager who feels defeated and crushed by life. She refuses to look the interviewer in the face. She constantly wrings her hands and sighs, 'I'm not worth all this time you're spending questioning me. Why don't you let me alone? Why can't I have the right to kill myself? I'm worthless and no good, so why waste precious time on me?'

After four months of psychotherapy Emily began to show a marked improvement in her attitude. Rapport was established between herself and the therapist. She began to talk freely of her childhood.

After six months of therapy Emily finally admitted the

real guilts which had been tormenting her. The following has been transcribed from her narrative:

'... I don't know why but I was glad my mother left Daddy for another man. I was seven at the time. I hated my mother and I felt ashamed because I hated her. She and I had never got along well. She always nagged me. I, my younger sister, and Daddy moved to a smaller apartment.

'I started keeping house for Daddy and we got along swell. We were very happy then. My Daddy used to make me feel like the most important girl in the world and I used to cook all sorts of things for supper which surprised him a whole lot. He told me that someday when I was older that maybe he'd marry me. I guess he meant it as a compliment or maybe he was putting me on, but at the time I took him very seriously. When I was twelve I got very sick and Daddy made me get into bed with him because I was crying and it comforted me to have him next to me. I think I had the flu or something like that. Anyway, we were very close then and I snuggled up against him and put my arms around him and I'd pretend that I was married to him. When I was well a few days later, I surprised Daddy by bringing him breakfast in bed on a Sunday morning. He hugged me and kissed me on the lips. I was in seventh heaven and I swear I felt important and great – just like I was really married to him. I wanted to make him happy; to make up to him for all those unhappy years he had spent being married to my mother.

'Then Daddy brought his woman home and she started to mind our business and boss us around. I hated her and I guess I showed it plenty because Daddy took a stand on her side and told me that unless I started treating her with respect he would make me regret acting the way I was. A few weeks later Daddy married her. She was strict and she made us go to church. I didn't want to go at first, but after awhile I started to go regularly and pretty soon I was head of the bible class.

'One day this preacher came to church and he gave this

sermon that upset me a great deal. He told all about incest and the crime of lust for one's own flesh and blood and he said that any such folks who lust for their own family is doomed to burn forever in hell. I got to thinking about this and I knew he was right – I had lusted for my own father and I had been glad my real mother had left home so I could have my own father all to myself. I started to worry about this and I guess I realized that I had sinned and I was worthless and no good and a harlot.'

Although Emily R.'s concept of 'lust' and her opinion of herself as a 'harlot' and 'sinful girl' were erroneous, nevertheless the feelings of self-loathing were quite real to herself. These feelings of guilt helped trigger her defeatist tendencies. Due to her earlier hostile relationship with her natural mother the stage had already been set within the theater of her immature mind. She henceforth decided to martyr herself. Other unconscious guilts and defense mechanisms were revealed as therapy progressed. She felt herself to blame because her father had 'sinned' also as the result of having 'slept' with her. Her concept of a sexual relationship with her father, except for an imagined one, was wholly altruistic in nature, yet she did not know this. To her way of thinking she was the 'seduced', but at the same time she believed she was the 'seducer' of her father because she had pretended, in her little girl's mind, to be her father's 'wife'. Thus, she felt she deserved to die. She decided to commit suicide because it was the only way to repent for her imagined 'sins'.

As the victim of an unwitting seduction, which was certainly entirely innocent in nature, Emily R. became obsessed with her guilt, withdrew from society, and became a potential suicide. Of course the 'sermon' she had heard had helped but eventually she would have convicted herself for her 'sins' anyway since she was certain she was guilty of 'incest' because she had nurtured licentious thoughts about her father.

This example of an unwitting 'seduction' is but one of many similar such occurrences taking place throughout the civilized world today. Children are prone to misconstrue their normal biological urges for 'sinful lustings' and therefore accept or rebel against their anxieties which arise because of it. Little do they seem to realize that they are thinking, feeling, and behaving normally. It is normal for the average child to desire the parent of the opposite sex during formative stages of early life. With the advent of maturity, these incestuous wishes disappear and become more socially acceptable in nature. The case in point is the little girl who prefers the society of other little girls to those of boys and vice versa – until puberty. Then the homosexual nature of their relationships change. Seduction in whatever form it occurs is both dangerous and unhealthy to the emotionally dependent, insecure, or maladjusted child, no matter how unintentional it might be.

Karen L. is a young lady of twenty-two who at the time this book was being written was serving a five year sentence in prison after being convicted for the second time for prostitution. Here is excerpted material from her case history:

Case No. 425
Karen L. Age 22
Committed for five years to the women's state reformatory, 2nd offense for prostitution.

' . . . My old lady and I never did get along. No wonder my old man deserted us when I was just a couple of years old. I hated her as long as I could remember and I used to do everything I could to needle her. Our relationship got better when I was about thirteen. She had this boy-friend, Mack. He was younger than her but handsome as hell and I couldn't see what he saw in my old lady except maybe that she was good in bed and she had a sexy figure.

'Anyway, Mack used to come around the house a lot and he used to be good to me. I guess I had a schoolgirl crush on him at first. Then we got pretty chummy and he used to tell me that he wouldn't marry my mother and would wait for me to get older. This got me all hot and bothered and I used to dream about taking him away from my old lady and marrying him. I used to ask him all kinds of things, like if I was sexy enough and stuff like that. He told me to take off my clothes and I did and he laughed and told me that I'd have to ripen some more before he could get interested. He said my old lady was really stacked and she knew how to perform in bed and that I ought to watch them in action.

'Well, I peeked in the keyhole one night and I saw them in bed. That excited me and at the same time it scared me, but I was determined to get him away from my mother. I used to masturbate sometimes thinking of us making love.

'One day when my old lady was working late Mack came around and I put on my sexiest robe and went into the living room where he was drinking beer and watching TV. I sat on his lap and he started feeling me. I was ready for him in any way he wanted me, but he smacked me on the behind with his hand and told me to come back when I knew what the score was.

'He must've told my old lady that I had been walking around with just a robe on and the old lady and me, we had it out. I got dressed and ran away. I got picked up by this truck driver and he was my first lover. It hurt something awful and I didn't come home for a couple of weeks. When I did the truant officer and the cops gave me a rough time. I confessed everything to Mack, like the stupid kid I was and I told him I did it all for him. He laughed and swore he was kidding. I hated him for putting me on like that and I decided to bust up the affair my mother was having with him. I got a condom and unwrapped it and put it in my bed where I was sure my old lady would find it. She did and I lied to her and told her that Mack had been my lover.

'She threw Mack out. She was pretty sweet to me after that for awhile, but then she got nasty again when she got this other guy to start coming around the house. His name was Willie. He was goodlooking and had a real manly phsyique. I cozied up to him and he laughed and pretended he was interested, but I was too young for him.

'I became more determined than ever to steal him away from my old lady. Finally I seduced him. He was easy on me and he liked me. One night he came around early and we started smooching and undressing each other. I was about fifteen at the time and I got so I enjoyed sex. My old lady had called the house and said she would be home at eight o'clock instead of at ten. I decided not to tell Willie that she was coming home early. We were in bed going at it real hot and heavy when my old lady came in. She caught us and threw us both the hell out.

'Willie felt sorry for me and he took me to live at his trailer. He worked for the race track as an exercise boy and we got along real sweet. He had a bum run of luck and I met a guy who offered me money. I liked being propositioned and I accepted. He took me to other guys and I started hustling professionally. You know the rest. They caught me several times and the last time the judge tossed me in the clink for five years. I'll bet if he could have been alone with me for a while he wouldn't have sent me up'.

The examining psychologist stated: 'Karen L. is a highly neurotic young lady with strong antisocial tendencies. She inwardly feels guilty for hating her mother. She loathes herself for having seduced her mother's boy friends [though it probably was the other way around]. Actually it was her mother who had enticed the child to become wanton through her own unmoral behavior and licentious activities in the house. At the time she first imagined she seduced Mack at age thirteen, if this man had been a responsible, upright individual, he could have discouraged her and instead encouraged her to remain in school and get a good education and give herself time in which to mature. Instead he foolishly – but *un*intentionally – seduced her for the first time by making a promise that he might marry her and that he would wait for her. In her immature mind that so eagerly wished for escape from an unhappy environment, she grasped this jokingly stated 'promise' as the real thing, misconstrued it for what it was, then set out to seduce Mack and steal him away from the mother she detested. The hate of her mother and the conflict between them was – and still is – a source of unconscious conflict in this young subject's mind. Long term psychotherapy and occupational rehabilitation is urgently needed.

At the time this book goes to press Karen L. is still in prison receiving punishment instead of the treatment she so desperately requires.

Unintentional seduction of children is a gravely serious problem because, more often than not, their immature minds are ready, willing, and able to grasp the wrong meanings from the words, actions, and gestures of the adults around them. These brief case histories reveal only a small portion of the problem and show just a few examples of what happens when children are unwittingly seduced. Children need understanding and instruction, not irresponsible enticement. The world of the child is vastly different from that of the adult. The child cannot communicate with the adult world. He or she must be encouraged to follow healthy pursuits rather than unhealthy ones. Most importantly, parents, teachers, clergymen, and other adults who come into contact with children must understand that unintentional seduction by innuendo, words, and so forth must be guarded against. The fire and brimstone harum-scarum of an irresponsible sermon can likewise seduce a child into believing he has 'sinned' against nature, and hence develop a guilt-ridden conscience. When the adult of today realizes that the child of today has sexual urges too, perhaps then more caution will be exercised in relationships with children.

Seduction in Childhood: Deliberate Seduction

THE DAMAGE done to the psychological makeup of an immature child who has been deliberately seduced by an adult or an older child is often irreparable. During normal development the child's understanding of life and love gradually evolves until puberty and finally, adulthood, are reached. Then he or she is capable emotionally and intellectually to cope with the realities of life. However, when gross sexuality is foisted upon an immature child whose intellect and emotional stability are undeveloped, a fixation often occurs. The child is most susceptible to the influence of adults and older children before puberty is reached. Hence, when a traumatic experience is foisted upon the immature mind, the child may react in a number of ways commensurate with his or her personality.

For instance, a little girl who has been seduced by an elder brother or perhaps a blood relative or neighbor, may become a wanton nymphet who uses her sexuality to taunt boys and men whom she knows, or she may become an introvert who displays a fear of males. She may display signs of hostility or even docility. She may become neurotic or even sociopathic. She may harbor feelings of guilt which may in turn cause her untold anguish which in turn may become symptomatic of emotional or mental illness. She many not suffer at all outwardly, but inwardly she may carry her guilt or shame or pangs of conscience as a badge of sin, affecting her entire outlook on life and no doubt stunting her normal psychological growth. Knowledge of licentious sexuality at too early an age is just as damaging to the psyche as drug addition is harmful. The sexuality experienced may become a child's obsession which may never be outgrown for the rest of his or her life.

Any physician who practices general medicine will admit, however reluctantly, that sexual relationships between adults and children of a statutory rape character occur more frequently than any other form of aberrant behavior. The general public does not hear of this for a number of reasons. In most cases the authorities never learn of such occurrences because the child is afraid to tell. In the majority of cases where such carnality has occurred, criminal charges are not pressed against the adult or teenage culprits. In those cases which are a matter for the courts to investigate and prosecute, the general public is usually unaware of such proceedings. The court shields the minor child from notoriety and publicity. The hearings are usually conducted in the privacy of the judges' chambers.

Occasionally the public does read of the arrest and conviction of a pedophile [child molester] who is sentenced for his crimes. However the general public does *not* learn of the countless others who go free because the children are afraid to tell what happened, or because they were victimized by close relatives. The shocking statistics dealing with the numbers of incestuous relationships between minor children and their close relatives may never be known, but the fact remains that incest is a common occurrence. Such relationships are totally destructive to the emotional stability of most children who are victims of such seductions. The following case histories bear out this appalling truth.

Case No. 1205
Eva W. Age 14
Subject was found to be six months' pregnant when examined by welfare clinic physician. Subject was impregnated by her stepfather who deserted family when pregnancy

became known. At time of interview subject was making baby clothes for her unborn infant in the county home for unwed mothers and appeared to be enjoying her sojourn like a child on a holiday. As the interview progressed it became evident to the psychiatric case worker that subject was sensitive and deeply troubled. Her joviality was a mask for her inner distress. A transcription of a tape recorded interview accompanies this abstract.

' . . . I'm really sorry for what happened. I wish I never would have done what I did. My stepfather always treated me nicely and he never raised a hand to me. He worked days and my mother worked nights in the bowling alley where she cashiers. He used to come home and help me with the dishes after we had supper and he was a good father to my younger sisters and little brother. One time when I was eleven he called me into his bedroom and asked me to rub his back. I did it and he said I was getting him all excited. I didn't know what he meant by that and I asked him. He had his shorts off. He turned over on his back and pulled down the sheet and showed me his penis. It made me blush to see him and he grabbed me and made me put my hand on it. Then he told me he'd beat hell out of me if I told mama.

'I didn't tell my mother and a couple of weeks later he did it again. He told me I was helping him out of his misery because it ached when it was erect and he showed me how to rub it with my hands. I was afraid when he started moaning and when it was over the sperm was all over my hands. I started to cry and he told me it was all right and he made me promise not to tell. He said he'd kill me if I told anybody and I was afraid so I didn't say anything.

'One Saturday he came home in the morning and gave my sisters and brother money to go to the movies. He told me to stay home because he wanted to see me alone. My mother was working and I was afraid of him so I ran out of the house when he went to drive the little kids to the

108

movie. He saw me running down the street. He stopped the car and slapped me and told me that I'd better come home and no buts about it.

'I did like he said and we went in the house and up to the bedroom. He took off all my clothes and then he took off his clothes and he started to kiss me all over. Pretty soon he started to ask me if it felt good and I said yes. He was glad and he kissed me on the mouth. I let him rub me between my legs and it felt wonderful. He told me that he loved me and he was wishing he was married to me instead of to mama. I told him he was joshing and he said he really meant it. I guess I liked what he was doing to me because I used to let him touch me down there everytime he wanted to after that.

'When I was twelve and started to have my monthlies he told me that I was now ripe and would soon be able to satisfy him like a real woman. It scared me to think of that big thing going inside me but he showed me with his fingers how I could stretch. He stretched me a lot of times with his fingers and it got me all hot and bothered. One day he put it in and he pulled me over on top of him and I did all the work. He laughed and said that I was a regular little nymphomaniac and he was glad he had taught me all about sex.

'A little while after that, he did it to me and fell asleep. I guess that's when he made me pregnant. When I missed my monthlies he got very worried and then one day he told me that he was going to kill me if I told on him. I started to cry and he slapped me and kicked me in the belly. I couldn't understand why he was treating me so bad and then when mama came home and saw the bruise on my face she wanted to know what had happened. He came in and said I had been bumming around with some boys and that I might be knocked up. Mama and him had a terrible fight and then he packed a suitcase, took all of our money and drove away in our car. When I started to get big and couldn't hide my belly, mama guessed the truth and brought me to the clinic. I was six months' gone. The doctor said she ought to swear out a warrant for my stepfather but she wouldn't do it. We don't know where he is at now. I hope I never see him again. I want to keep my baby after it's born, but they say I got to give it away for adoption. I'll die if they make me do that. Why can't I keep my baby?'

Similar case histories are taken every day throughout the land. Regardless of the outcome, young girls like Eva will never be the same again. Not only have been robbed of a normal childhood, but they suffer an irreparable psychological trauma from which there is no recovery. The deliberate seduction of children by malicious adults is the most heartless of all individual crimes that can be inflicted – especially when it is a case of incest.

The seduction of young children by adult women is not quite so prevalent in occurrence as that perpetrated by adult males; however it does occur with alarming frequency. The following case history is typical.

Case No. 240
Charles A. Age 16
Subject was placed in a foster home after his maternal mother was sentenced to one year in the woman's reformatory for contributing to the delinquency of a minor. Psychiatric case worker interviewed the subject regularly twice weekly for a period of seven months before rapport was established and the truth of what had taken place was admitted. At first he refused to 'rat' on his mother. But when he was able to realize that he was suffering emotionally because of the relationship he had had with his delinquent mother, he finally confessed what had taken place. The following is a transcript of his statement.

' . . . Maybe I am more upset about what my mother and I used to do than I thought. It bothered me, I guess,

110

but I didn't really face up to it until now. Now that you mention it, I suppose I do know that what we used to do was wrong and I felt secretly ashamed of it.

'My father was killed in the Korean War when I was only a couple of years old. My mother took it pretty bad and I guess she cracked up over it. She had this baby sitter take care of me while she worked. She worked as a stenographer in a big office building where there are a lot of lawyers. When I was eleven or twelve she changed jobs and went to work at night, working for some court reporters typing up stuff that had to be ready in the morning. That way she was home to see me off to school every morning. She would sleep while I was in school and would have dinner ready at night. She always was very close to me and was very possessive. She used to pick my friends and she didn't like me to have any girl friends.

'She used to hug and kiss me and tell me that she wanted to be my girl friend. She always said I looked just like my dad. Sometimes she used to show me his pictures and compare them with the way I looked.

'Whenever my mother had a day off from work we would go places together. She would give me money and I'd pay the check if we ate in a restaurant or I'd buy the tickets if we went to a movie. She never went out with any men on dates because she told me that she only wanted to be with me. When I was fourteen I had this party to go to and I was supposed to take a girl so when I told my mother she said that I ought not go unless I could take her since she was my girl. Then she said that she didn't go out on dates with men because I was her boy friend, so it was only right that I be "true" to her too.

'Well, that sounded logical so I didn't. She was very happy about that and I didn't go to that party. That night I went to bed and my mother came in and got in bed next to me. She hugged me and kissed me and asked me to put my arms around her. I did and I noticed that she was only wearing this real thin nightgown. I didn't think anything about it and I fell asleep.

111

'I woke up later on when I felt my mother pushing her hips against me. I pretended I was asleep and I noticed that she had her eyes closed too. It was dark in the room but there was enough light shining in the window to see her face. She put one of her legs around mine and rubbed against me. It felt very good and I continued to make out I was sleeping. Then she pushed my pajama pants down and played with my organ. I was pretty mature for my age and I already knew a whole lot about sex. and I didn't much care that it was my mother there in bed with me because I was so excited. When it was over I fell asleep and she was still half laying on me.

'After that time it happened a lot, sometimes every couple of nights when she wasn't working. One Sunday morning last year when I was fifteen we did it in the morning and she saw that I was awake and I saw that she was awake too. I guess we both had been pretending we were doing that in our sleep. I felt real ashamed.

'This guy I know used to tell me all sorts of things about sex and how he used to masturbate while watching his mother through the keyhole when she was undressed. His name is Joey and we were always very close buddies. I never talked much about myself and he was always real curious. He noticed how private I kept my own sex doings and he kept egging me on to tell him. He also noticed how protective my mother was of me and how possessive she was and all. One day he asked me some stuff about what I did when I got hardup and I refused to tell him. Then he called me a mother——. I turned real red in the face and he started teasing me and yelling that he was right and he knew it all the time. Then he said he'd tell everybody in the neighborhood and he started to run out. I grabbed him and begged him not to say anything. I shouldn't have said that because then he knew that he had guessed the truth.

'Okay, he promised he wouldn't say nothing *if* I would let him hide in the house somewhere and watch us. I was very nervous about it, but that was better than having him blab it all over the neighborhood. Joey was seventeen and he was a real creep when it came down to it and I guess I never really realized how much of a dirty so-and-so he was until that day. But he said he would only watch and nothing else would happen.

'That Sunday morning about eight o'clock, Joey sneaked into the house through a window I had left open for him. He sneaked over to the bedroom door which was open and was there when I woke up. My mother was sleeping with her back to me. I tried to signal him to hide himself better but my movements woke her up. She sat up and pulled her nightie off over her head. Then she started to kiss me. I felt real embarrassed and ashamed because I knew Joey was there watching us and she didn't. The sunlight shined in the window like a spotlight on the bed. My mother and I were making love for a long time. First she was on top and then me on top. Finally she finished and rolled over on her belly and went to sleep. I got out of bed and saw that Joey was gone.

'That evening just when my mother and I were sitting down in the kitchen to eat supper there was this loud knocking on the door. I went to open it and some cops came rushing in. They locked my mother up and they took me to the juvenile section.

'I found out that Joey had taken a polaroid camera when he had sneaked in that morning and had snapped a lot of pictures of us. He was showing them around to some of the kids on the block when a cop grabbed him. He was arrested for having dirty pictures. Then he ratted on us and that's the truth, so help me.'

This incredible but true case history had a tragic ending. Charles' mother committed suicide in the reformatory. She should not have been imprisoned for what she had done. She was a sick woman, emotionally unstable, and not responsible for her actions. She had killed herself because she had been unable to stand the constant taunting and harassment of her fellow inmates.

Charles had a serious emotional relapse following his mother's funeral. He is presently receiving out patient treatment at a mental hospital in another city. He has become backward in his schoolwork and suffers from a muscular tic in his face. The traumatic effect of the derision of his former friends and schoolmates plus the guilt for what he has done may permanently affect him.

A parallel to the case just presented is this one which did not end quite so tragically.

Case 926
Benjamin P. Age 19
Subject was arrested for lewd and lascivous behavior. He was picked up on the street masquerading as a woman. The following is the excerpted report filed by the psychiatric case worker who investigated the subject before judicial dispensation. The material was transcribed from the subject's own voluntary statements.

' . . . Ever since I was a small child my mother treated me like a girl. I was ten before she took me to a barber shop for a haircut. I used to have gorgeous long curls. My father never objected because he said I looked more feminine than masculine and he liked to see my mother happy. I took dancing lessons and studied the ballet. The teachers said I had the grace of a prima ballerina and I would go places if I pursued my studies. I was always extremely close with mother and she and I often went shopping together. I learned to cook and help her in the kitchen and I adored being like a daughter to her. I have a younger brother, but he treats my parents and me horribly. He's a little animal. Thank heavens he's away from the house. They accepted him in the military academy you know.
' . . . I never dated girls because it was not to my taste. Frankly, I always wished I was a girl and had female
114

sex organs. Mother said that perhaps someday I could have an operation. She said that my skin was not at all like a boy's and I'm inclined to agree, don't you think so too?' [No comment.]

'. . . Mother permitted me to dress like a girl around the house and I simply adored wearing her nylon panties and her garter belts. They felt so keen.

'I was about eighteen when I had my first crush. I fell head over heels for the most dashing young fellow you ever did see. But he wouldn't have anything to do with me. Then I met this sweet young chap who seemed interested in me. I suppose I submitted to him because I was on the rebound, just crushed from the rebuff, you know.

'I dressed in drag a few times and I felt positively wicked cruising. There were some marvelous kids who dug me the most and we hit it off just swell. When they arrested me I was never so mortified in all my life. I think it's positively outrageous. I was not committing a crime. Can I help it if I'm gay? My mother thinks it's an outrage too.'

In this case the subject identified with the maternal parent due to the total domination by his mother. As further interviews were conducted it was learned that the father had always 'treated' his son as a daughter. In this manner he 'seduced' his own son into believing he was homosexual. Later investigation revealed that the father of the subject was an overt homosexual who had encouraged the same behavior in his son. The mother, a domineering, shrewish woman, often suggested to her son that he was more attractive to males than she had been. He identified with her and subsequently became a homosexual. Had his father *not seduced* him, there might have been a chance for the subject to overcome [or possibly outgrow] his effeminate inclinations. There is no doubt in the psychiatrists' minds who examined the subject that he is a confirmed homosexual and transvestite [dressing or masquerading in the clothing of the opposite sex] and there is little hope that he will ever change.

115

Case 370
Joanne G. Age 12
Committed to home for wayward girls. Incorrigible behavior, chronic truancy, petty thefts, disobedience to parents and complete lack of regard for authority. The child's own parents had her committed since they were unable to control her.

Psychiatric case worker reported that Joanne is eldest of three siblings, a boy age ten and two twin girls, age eight, The parents are hardworking diligent people who maintain a neat home behind the gasoline station they operate in the suburbs of a large eastern city. The parents were at a loss to understand what had happened to Joanne and had tried to have her treated by psychologists, but the therapy was rejected. Joanne, a tall girl for her age looks much older than her years. She wears makeup heavily applied and is a chain smoker. Her attitude is vindictive and hostile. She slumps in her chair and glares defiantly when asked to stand up or to sit up straight.

After she was committed to the county home she was quick to vie for leadership of the other inmates, even girls three and four years her senior. She was confined without privileges for breaking the rules and after several months of punishment and denial of privileges [watching television, occupational therapy, etc.] she finally promised to cooperate with the psychiatrist.

Several months after the therapy began the heart of the problem was reached. The psychiatrist soon realized that he had discovered the real reason why twelve-year-old Joanne had become so incorrigible. Here is the transcript of her somewhat shocking statement:

'I guess you're right, doctor, about me acting like I was mad at the whole world. Maybe I am. I got a dirty deal and I guess I tried to make everybody I know pay for it. I didn't feel like anything and I wanted them all to sit up and notice me and say nice things about me. About this dirty deal I started to tell you about. You promise you won't say anything about it to my mother?'

[At this point the psychiatrist asked: 'Why?']

'Maybe it's because I really don't want her to know. I think that maybe it would kill her if she found out about my uncle and me. That's her brother, Uncle Kenny.

'. . . I think I was around six years old then when Uncle Kenny came around the house to stay with us for a while. He was going to college and was going to be a big shot in agriculture. He was very good looking and I loved him something fierce. I always was one to speak my mind, even at that age, and I told him that I wanted to marry him. The whole family thought that was real funny and my mother said that I could never marry Uncle Kenny because that would be incest, which is being married to your blood kin, which is a sin against God.

'Uncle Kenny took me real serious and he said he loved me too. He brought me presents – gave me a real expensive doll once – and he took me for long walks in the woods behind our house.

'One time we went to this swimming hole and nobody was there and Uncle Kenny said we could go swimming if I promised not to tell. I was very thrilled and we got undressed and went swimming. We didn't have no towels so we laid on the ground in the sun to get dry. Uncle Kenny showed me his thing and told me to kiss it to prove that I loved him. I did and he then played with me. It was very large and I liked to take it in my mouth.

'After that we played around everytime we were alone and he gave me all sorts of presents and then, when he was going to go back to school, he gave me a real engagement ring from the dime store. I cried and he told me to keep our engagement secret.

'I did keep the secret. He came back and stayed at our house very often and nobody suspected a thing. My folks always had to tend to business so we were alone a lot and we did a lot of sexy things. I got so I couldn't wait for him to come home and he always brought me a present.

Pretty soon I began to believe that someday we both would really get married to each other.

'When I was eleven – it was two days after my birthday – my mother and father told me that Uncle Kenny was getting married. I didn't believe them and I stole some money from the cash register and took a bus to the town where Uncle Kenny lived near where he was going to the agriculture college. He was real surprised to see me and he didn't answer me when I asked him if he was really going to get married to someone else. We got in bed and I did all sorts of things to him, even some things I had never done before. Then his telephone rang and it was the girl he was going to marry.

'My heart was broken because he lied to me. I ran away and some cops found me and they called my folks who came and got me. I never told them about me and Uncle Kenny. I just felt worthless and no good and I remembered what my mother had said about incest and I was worried about that. I hated my uncle and I hated my mother and I hated everybody. I wanted everybody to like me and pay attention to me, I guess, so I did all kinds of bad things. I wanted to show the world that I wasn't afraid of nobody and that I was just as good as the next person.'

This was only the beginning of Joanne's psychotherapy. At the present she is showing progress, but several years of intensive psychotherapy is still required to correct her attitude toward life and to overcome the harm that her foolish and immature uncle has done to her. She will bear the psychological scars for life of the wantonly deliberate seduction. But perhaps she is one of the fortunate little girls after all because psychological help is being given to her. Too often other children who have been victimized by adult seducers carry their burdens of guilt throughout life and never recover as a result.

Case No. 1610
Lisa P. Age 14

Subject was arrested while burglarizing a house with three young men aged 21, 25, and 26. She was taken to the juvenile detention home where a psychiatric examination and psychological evaluation tests were made. Subject was paroled in the custody of her parents on the condition that psychiatric therapy by a private psychiatrist be given. Eight months later the following report was tendered to the juvenile court judge by the therapist:

'Lisa responded to therapy rapidly. She had made excellent progress and it is doubtful that she will repeat her delinquent behavior. She is the youngest of two siblings. Another child, a sister, was stillborn. Her living sister works for a food processing company as a packer. Her parents get along nicely and their relationship with Lisa is good. Father works as a long-distance truck driver. Mother is employed as a checker in a supermarket. Additional income is earned by the family from rent collected from roomers, a man and a woman who reside in the two upstairs bedrooms.

'At age eleven Lisa was encouraged to go for a ride with some older boys, provided she "proved" she was a good sport. She enjoyed this attention and gladly permitted them to fondle and kiss her. There was no sexual contact at that time. She felt wanted and superior because she was allowed to accompany the boys. The gang leader encouraged her to be "his girl". He taught her to commit fellatio which she performed on him and subsequently, the other boys. Later the gang was arrested for auto larceny and she did not see them again until after they had served their time. She was encouraged to accompany them on their burglaries and often served as lookout. She had been seduced into believing that the gang leader, age twenty-six, was in love with her and that he was only stealing in order to save up enough for a "nest egg" which would enable them to run away and get married.

119

'Lisa now realizes she had been duped. There are some guilt feelings about her past sexual activities but she is rapidly learning to dispel them and not blame herself. She is of high intelligence and has the ability to work diligently. Since therapy has begun she has shown remarkable progress in her schoolwork and has a "B" average. Her only worry is that someday when she does marry, she may lose the love of her husband when he learns she is not a virgin. In time, this fear too may be overcome.'

Case No. 843–NY
Peggy D. Age 17
Subject was apprehended near the scene of a deliberately set fire in which a man, age 61 perished. She was turned over to the juvenile authorities and charged with arson. She was sentenced to the state mental hospital to receive therapy which the examing psychiatrists believed was needed. The following is a transcript of statements subject made during subsequent examinations:

'... I can't lie to you anymore. I've got to get this thing off my chest and I've got to tell somebody and because you really are trying to help me, Doctor, I might as well get it over with. Sure, I set that fire. I had thought about it for a long time and I couldn't put it off any longer. Ed, that's the man who died in the fire, I knew him for a long time. For two years to be exact. He used to be out in his yard raking up the leaves when I would walk by on my way home from school. He always said nice things and complimented me and I guess I lapped it up. He said I was very beautiful and that I ought to be a model. I said he was joshing me but he insisted that he was telling the truth. Then he told me he was a photographer and he'd like to take some glamour pictures of me, some of which he'd give me if I posed for him. I said I wasn't interested, but then he offered me money.

'I thought about it and one day I agreed to go inside his house with him and pose for a dollar an hour. He was very nice and he treated me like a queen. He used to have me over twice a week and he would give me three dollars every time I came over. I got along very nicely with him, and I got to enjoy his company – and I guess, trust him, too. That was my mistake. He talked me into posing in bikinis, then later, I started posing naked.

'One day when I was holding a pose he seemed to be taking an unusually long time in snapping my picture. I stepped down from the pedestal when I didn't see him behind his camera on the tripod and called out to him. He said he was in the darkroom and for me to come in he wanted to show me something. I went over and opened the door, covering myself with a big towel. The lights were off and it was black as pitch in there and he said for me to come in and quickly close the door. I did and then he grabbed me and kissed me and said he loved me. I was frightened because he had yanked the towel off and I had the feeling that he was naked too. I slapped him and ran out and he ran after me. He was nude and he said that unless I let him make love to me that he would publish my naked pictures in a magazine and my parents would find out. I begged him not to do that and he said he wouldn't if I promised to let him make love to me. I said I was afraid because I was a virgin and he said he wouldn't take my virginity away. I made him promise that and he swore that he wouldn't. Then he turned the lights down real low and I lay down on a couch and he kissed me all over from the top of my head to my toes. It was wonderful the way he kissed and he told me he loved me and that was why it was so wonderful to me. I guess I got to enjoy that kind of kissing and I used to think about it and the way he tongued me. It drove me half out of my mind and it got so that I was dropping in to let him kiss me down there like that every day.

'Well, about six months ago I met a boy that I was very attracted to. He is a year older than me, a senior in high school. We started dating and pretty soon were steadies. I never would let him touch me down there even if he tried – which he didn't because he's too much of a gentleman for that and he respects me too much. I started to think about Ed and I decided that it was time I called a halt to what I was doing with him, although I didn't do anything but lay still while he kissed me. I started to worry about this because I'd heard it wasn't natural. They call it cunnilingus and it's supposed to be a perversion when it's indulged in exclusively. I began to think that maybe Ed was turning me into a pervert. It worried me a lot. Then one Friday night my boy friend and I were coming out of a movie when we bumped into Ed. He looked at me very peculiarly and I got upset. Nothing was said and we walked away and he walked away. My boy friend and I drove out in the park and we sat in the car for awhile. We were necking and I got very hot and bothered and I wanted him to do what Ed had done to me and I was afraid to ask him. I think I wanted that more than anything. But my boy friend didn't try anything and we went home.

'The next day, Saturday morning, the phone rang. It was Ed. He told me to come over right away – or else. His tone of voice scared me. I went over and he accused me of letting my boy friend eat me too. I called him a filthy old man and I ran out. He yelled after me that he would publish those pictures. I turned around and went back in the house and I ran all through the rooms searching for the pictures with Ed following me. He said he had the pictures and the negatives hidden and he wouldn't give them up ever.

'I begged him to let me go but he said he wouldn't and he grabbed me and got down on his knees and pulled my dress up. I pushed him away and ran out. I was afraid I would never get away from him – unless he was dead. I wished I could find those negatives and prints and I wished I could burn them up. Then I hit on the idea of burning down Ed's house and getting rid of the pictures

122

at the same time. Then I would be free of him. I got some gasoline and hid it under his porch. But a long time went by before I got up nerve to do it. A couple of months after I had hid the gas under his porch, I made up my mind it was then or never. But I still couldn't get up nerve enough to do it. So I decided to give up the idea when a terrible thing happened. Ed sent a nude picture of me to my boy friend. He mailed it to him, and God knows how his parents didn't see it. Anyway, my boy friend showed it to me the night he got it and asked what it was all about. I blushed something awful and told him I didn't know – that it really wasn't me – that maybe one of the jealous girls who also wanted to date him had taken a picture of my head and pasted it on the naked body. Before he could examine the picture, I snatched it out of his hands and ripped it up and then I burned up the pieces.

'It was around midnight that night when I sneaked over to Ed's and knocked on his door. I asked him why he had sent my boy friend that picture and he laughed and said he would do that to all my boy friends, and my parents too. Then he told me to take off my clothes and lay on the bed. I wouldn't. He pushed me down and pulled off my panties, then he got down between my thighs and went at me like a wild animal. He played with himself at the same time and it was so disgusting that I wanted to puke. Finally he got it over with and went to sleep with his head between my legs. I got out of bed, went outside quietly, took the gas can and spilled it all over the house. Then I lit a match, dropped it on the floor and ran out.

'The streets were deserted at that hour and the police saw me running away from the blazing house. They smelled gasoline on my clothes where I accidentally spilled some when I was dumping the stuff on the floors and over the furniture. You know the rest. I'm sorry for what happened.'

The court remanded Peggy to the state mental hospital because it was learned that the sixty-one year old man who had seduced her and later blackmailed her into submitting to his lewd advances had a long police record of similar offenses against underage girls. It was also learned that two other girls in the neighbourhood were also being seduced in the same manner. The psychiatric case worker's findings indicated that Peggy would recover from her emotional dilemma if the state gave her the chance. At this writing she is recovering from the trauma and is expected to return to society before her twentieth birthday.

Only a few of the numerous types of seduction dangers have been illustrated in this chapter. It is hoped that these sufficiently point out the harmful after affects of childhood seduction. It is obvious that the child victim's emotions and mind can be crippled for life when sexual seduction is committed at this early age.

*   *   *

The seduction art has its dangers and its delights. But above all, remember it is *love* which satisfies the hungers of the body. Man must have mental peace of mind if he is to be truly secure in his physical life as well.

Lovemaking is to the seduction art what vitamins are to healthy life. When two lovers show their feelings without inhibition and shame, and do not deny each other the richness of their understanding and compassionate love, the seduction art becomes second nature to them because it is 'doing what comes naturally.'

THE END

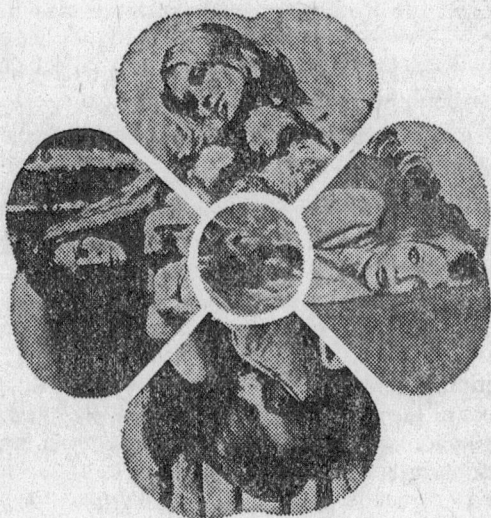

Crazy New Year '71
The pleasure of your pleasure
is requested by
Simone.. Anita.. Lou.. Beverley

The Crazy Ladies

...not forgetting Robert Fingerhood,
super sex star

8s. (40p) paperback

NEL BESTSELLERS

Crime

F.2773	THE LIGHT OF DAY	Eric Ambler 5/-
F.2786	ABILITY TO KILL	Eric Ambler 5/-
F.2574	MURDER CAME LATE	John Creasey 5/-
F.2445	SAMANTHA	E. V. Cunningham 5/-
F.2446	ALICE	E. V. Cunningham 5/-
F.2447	PHYLLIS	E. V. Cunningham 5/-
F.2799	THE MURDER LEAGUE	Robert L. Fish 6/-
F.2365	TICKET TO DEATH	Ed. McBain 5/-
F.2876	MURDER MUST ADVERTISE	Dorothy L. Sayers 7/-
F.2849	STRONG POISON	Dorothy L. Sayers 6/-
F.2897	IN THE TEETH OF THE EVIDENCE	Dorothy L. Sayers 7/-
F.2848	CLOUDS OF WITNESS	Dorothy L. Sayers 6/-
F.2845	THE DOCUMENTS IN THE CASE	Dorothy L. Sayers 6/-
F.2877	WHOSE BODY?	Dorothy L. Sayers 6/-
F.2749	THE NINE TAILORS	Dorothy L. Sayers 6/-
F.2871	THE UNPLEASANTNESS AT THE BELLONA CLUB	Dorothy L. Sayers 6/-
F.2750	FIVE RED HERRINGS	Dorothy L. Sayers 6/-
F.2826	UNNATURAL DEATH	Dorothy L. Sayers 6/-
F.2870	BLOODY MAMA	Robert Thom 5/-
F.2629	THE CON GAME	Hillary Waugh 5/-

Fiction

F.2755	PAID SERVANT	E. R. Braithwaite 6/-
F.2289	THE SPANISH GARDENER	A. J. Cronin 5/-
F.2261	THE CITADEL	A. J. Cronin 7/6
F.2318	THE KEYS OF THE KINGDOM	A. J. Cronin 7/6
F.2752	THE HARRAD EXPERIMENT	Robert H. Rimmer 6/-
F.2920	PROPOSITION 31	Robert H. Rimmer 6/-
F.2427	THE ZOLOTOV AFFAIR	Robert H. Rimmer 6/-
F.2704	THE REBELLION OF YALE MARRATT	Robert H. Rimmer 6/-
F.2896	THE CARPETBAGGERS	Harold Robbins 15/-
F.2918	THE ADVENTURERS	Harold Robbins 15/-
F.2657	A STONE FOR DANNY FISHER	Harold Robbins 8/-
F.2654	NEVER LOVE A STRANGER	Harold Robbins 12/-
F.2653	THE DREAM MERCHANTS	Harold Robbins 12/-
F.2917	WHERE LOVE HAS GONE	Harold Robbins 12/-
F.2155	NEVER LEAVE ME	Harold Robbins 5/-
F.2580	THE BEAUTIFUL COUPLE	William Woolfolk 7/6
F.2327	THE SERPENT AND THE STAFF	Frank Yerby 7/6
F.2479	AN ODOUR OF SANCTITY	Frank Yerby 10/-
F.2326	BENTON'S ROW	Frank Yerby 7/6
F.2822	GILLIAN	Frank Yerby 8/-
F.2895	CAPTAIN REBEL	Frank Yerby 6/-
F.2421	THE VIXENS	Frank Yerby 7/6
F.2143	A WOMAN CALLED FANCY	Frank Yerby 5/-
F.2223	THE OLD GODS LAUGH	Frank Yerby 5/-

Romance

F.2500	GIFT OF THE DESERT	Hermina Black 5/-
F.2501	GOLD MOON OF AFRICA	Hermina Black 5/-
F.2502	THE MARRIAGE OF SUSAN	Hermina Black 5/-
F.2351	THE BEAUTY SURGEON	Ursula Bloom 4/-
F.2352	CASUALTY WARD	Ursula Bloom 4/-
F.2577	DOCTOR'S DESIRE	Ursula Bloom 4/-
F.2578	NURSE JUDY'S SECRET PASSION	Ursula Bloom 4/-
F.2152	TWO LOVES	Denise Robins 3/6
F.2153	THE PRICE OF FOLLY	Denise Robins 3/6
F.2154	WHEN A WOMAN LOVES	Denise Robins 3/6
F.2241	THIS IS LOVE	Denise Robins 3/6
F.2563	RETURN OF A SOLDIER	Rebecca West 4/-

Science Fiction

F.2658	GLORY ROAD	Robert Heinlein 7/6
F.2844	STRANGER IN A STRANGE LAND	Robert Heinlein 12/-
F.2630	THE MAN WHO SOLD THE MOON	Robert Heinlein 6/-
F.2386	PODKAYNE OF MARS	Robert Heinlein 6/-
F.2449	THE MOON IS A HARSH MISTRESS	Robert Heinlein 8/-
F.2754	DUNE	Frank Herbert 12/-

War

F.2695	THE MAN THEY COULDN'T KILL	Dennis Holman 5/-
F.2484	THE FLEET THAT HAD TO DIE	Richard Hough 5/-
F.2805	HUNTING OF FORCE Z	Richard Hough 5/-
F.2494	P.Q.17—CONVOY TO HELL	Lund Ludlam 5/-
F.2423	STRIKE FROM THE SKY—THE BATTLE OF BRITAIN STORY	
		Alexander McKee 6/-
F.2471	THE STEEL COCOON	Bentz Plagemann 5/-
F.2645	THE LONGEST DAY	Cornelius Ryan 5/-
F.2146	THE LAST BATTLE (illustrated)	Cornelius Ryan 12/6

Western

Walt Slade—Bestsellers

F.2506	LEAD AND FLAME	Bradford Scott 4/-
F.2634	THE SKY RIDERS	Bradford Scott 4/-
F.2648	OUTLAW ROUNDUP	Bradford Scott 4/-
F.2649	RED ROAD TO VENGEANCE	Bradford Scott 4/-
F.2669	BOOM TOWN	Bradford Scott 4/-
F.2687	THE RIVER RAIDERS	Bradford Scott 4/-

General

F.2721	EROTIC EDWARDIAN FAIRY TALES	Anon. 6/-
F.2420	THE SECOND SEX	Simone De Beauvoir 8/6
F.2234	SEX MANNERS FOR MEN	Robert Chartham 5/-
F.2531	SEX MANNERS FOR ADVANCED LOVERS	Robert Chartham 5/-
F.2766	SEX MANNERS FOR THE YOUNG GENERATION	Robert Chartham 5/-
F.2374	SEX WITHOUT GUILT	Albert Ellis Ph.D. 8/6
U.2366	AN ABZ OF LOVE	Inge and Sten Hegeler 10/6
U.2851	A HAPPIER SEX LIFE (illustrated)	Dr. Sha Kokken 12/-
F.2136	WOMEN	John Philip Lundin 5/-
F.2333	MISTRESSES	John Philip Lundin 5/-
F.2511	SEXUALIS '95	Jacques Sternberg 5/-
F.2720	THE FIRST TIME	Paul Tabori 6/-
F.2584	SEX MANNERS FOR SINGLE GIRLS	Dr. G. Valensin 5/-
F.2592	THE FRENCH ART OF SEX MANNERS	Dr. G. Valensin 5/-

Mad

S.3702	A MAD LOOK AT OLD MOVIES	5/-
S.3523	BOILING MAD	5/-
S.3496	THE MAD ADVENTURES OF CAPTAIN KLUTZ	5/-
S.3719	THE QUESTIONABLE MAD	5/-
S.3714	FIGHTING MAD	5/-
S.3613	HOWLING MAD	5/-
S.3477	INDIGESTIBLE MAD	5/-

— —

NEL P.O. BOX 11, FALMOUTH, CORNWALL

Please send cheque or postal order. Allow 9d. per book to cover postage and packing (Overseas 1/- per book).

Name..

Address ....

....

Title ....
(AUGUST)